CARPAL FRACTURE-DISLOCATIONS

EDITED BY

THOMAS E. TRUMBLE, MD
PROFESSOR AND CHIEF
HAND AND MICROVASCULAR SURGERY SERVICE
UNIVERSITY OF WASHINGTON MEDICAL CENTER
SEATTLE, WASHINGTON

SERIES EDITOR

THOMAS R. JOHNSON, MD

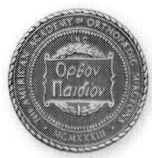

American Academy of Orthopaedic Surgeons

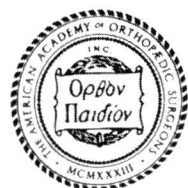

American Academy of Orthopaedic Surgeons
6300 North River Road
Rosemont, IL 60018
1-800-626-6726

The American Academy of Orthopaedic Surgeons Monograph Series is dedicated to Wendy O. Schmidt, American Academy of Orthopaedic Surgeons senior medical editor, 1987-1991.

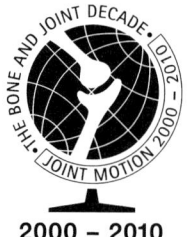

2000 – 2010

CONTRIBUTORS

Brian D. Adams, MD
Professor
Department of Orthopaedic Surgery
University of Iowa
Iowa City, Iowa

Christopher Allan, MD
Assistant Professor
Department of Orthopaedics
University of Washington
Seattle, Washington

Philip E. Blazar, MD
Instructor, Orthopaedic Surgery
Brigham and Women's Hospital
Harvard Medical School
Boston, Massachusetts

Evan D. Collins, MD
Assistant Professor
Department of Orthopedics
Baylor College of Medicine
Houston, Texas

Brian J. Divelbiss, MD
Dickson-Diveley Midwest Orthopaedic Clinic
Kansas City, Missouri

Eric P. Hofmeister, MD
Department of Orthopaedic Surgery
Naval Medical Center, San Diego
San Diego, California

Molly Hudson, OTR, CHT
The Woodlands Hand Rehabilitation Center
The Woodlands, Texas

Jeffrey N. Lawton, MD
Assistant Professor
Department of Orthopaedic Surgery
University of Kentucky
Lexington, Kentucky

L. Randall Mohler, MD
Department of Orthopaedic Surgery
Sharp Rees-Stealy Medical Group
San Diego, California

Peter M. Murray, MD
Senior Associate Consultant
Division of Hand and Microvascular Surgery
Department of Orthopaedic Surgery
The Mayo Clinic
Jacksonville, Florida

Alexander Y. Shin, MD
Director, Hand and Microvascular Surgery
Department of Orthopaedic Surgery
Naval Medical Center, San Diego
San Diego, California

Jade Strong, MOT, OTR, CHT
The Woodlands Hand Rehabilitation Center
The Woodlands, Texas

Matthew M. Tomaino, MD
Associate Professor
Department of Orthopaedic Surgery
University of Pittsburgh
Pittsburgh, Pennsylvania

Thomas E. Trumble, MD
Professor and Chief
Hand and Microvascular Surgery Service
Department of Orthopaedics and Sports Medicine
University of Washington Medical Center
Seattle, Washington

Duc P. Vo, MD
Orthopaedic Associates of Garland
Garland, Texas

CONTENTS

PREFACE

This monograph is written for all the surgeons taking trauma call who find themselves faced with the complex spectrum of fractures and dislocations of the carpus. I hope that the information provided here will enhance their ability to accurately diagnose and skillfully reconstruct these injuries, thereby helping patients regain flexibility and strength and avoid the pain of traumatic arthritis.

Our understanding of these complex injuries has increased as a result of the detailed clinical studies and innovative biomechanical research conducted by many of our colleagues over the years. Also, advances in medicine in the last decade allow surgeons today to offer improved diagnostic tests to pinpoint the area of injury and techniques to access bone blood supply. In addition, orthopaedic surgeons have researched and developed special devices, such as scaphoid screws and suture anchors, that facilitate anatomic reconstruction of the delicate, watchwork-like mechanism of the wrist.

I would like to recognize several incredible educators and surgeons who helped to train a generation of orthopaedic surgeons: The late Richard J. Smith, MD, founded the Hand Surgery Service at Massachusetts General Hospital and developed novel lessons to educate students of all ages. Wayne O. Southwick, MD, now Professor Emeritus at Yale University in the Department of Orthopaedics, always encouraged residents and faculty to consider how to treat patients not just for today but for the course of their lives. He stressed that patient function and symptoms should be given priority over radiographs and similar measurements. Jesse B. Jupiter, MD, who has taken over as Chief of the Hand Surgery Service at Massachusetts General Hospital after Dr. Smith passed away, and James R. Urbaniak, MD, Professor and Chairman of Orthopaedic Surgery at Duke University, are innovative surgeons who have led other orthopaedic surgeons to "think outside the box." They have proved that many challenges, such as microcirculation and restoration of joints, were not only theoretically but also practically solvable.

A surgeon's education never stops with a residency or fellowship. American Academy of Orthopaedic Surgeons (AAOS) courses and monographs such as this help us further our knowledge. We also continue to learn from our practice and our partners. I feel fortunate to be able to learn from a wonderful group of partners, including Christopher Allan, MD, Douglas Hanel, MD, John Sack, MD, and Nicholas Vedder, MD, who continue to set the bar high for treating hand injuries.

I also would like to acknowledge Laurie Braun, Associate Senior Editor at the AAOS, who has guided this project to produce a monograph of such high quality. Finally, I want to recognize Thomas Johnson, MD, Monograph Series Editor for the AAOS, who has led the effort to expand our knowledge base on complex orthopaedic issues that can be best addressed in a monograph format.

Thomas E. Trumble, MD

CHAPTER 1

ANATOMY OF THE WRIST LIGAMENTS

BRIAN D. ADAMS, MD
BRIAN J. DIVELBISS, MD

The wrist is a complex joint composed of 15 bones and a multitude of articulations. Motion occurs primarily at the radiocarpal and midcarpal joints, and stability is achieved by ligamentous restraint more than by bony congruence. Wrist ligament injuries are a common cause of pathologic instabilities, often resulting in pain, weakness, and stiffness. This chapter reviews the anatomy and function of the key wrist ligaments.

The nomenclature used for wrist ligaments varies, creating some confusion. The terms *intrinsic* and *extrinsic* have been used to differentiate ligaments that reside primarily within the joint from those that are located entirely within the outer capsule. Alternative and perhaps more anatomically descriptive terms are *interosseous* and *capsular*. Capsular ligaments are fibrous thickenings that reside within the capsule and contain collagen-filled bundles covered by a synovial lamina on the articular side and a fibrous lamina on the outside; many also contain neurovascular structures that contribute to the vascularity of the carpal bones. Interosseous ligaments lack a fibrous lamina and are located entirely within the joint. The terms *interosseous* and *capsular* are also more consistent with clinical practice, where the term *interosseous ligament* is typically used to describe the scapholunate and lunotriquetral ligaments, which are often the focus of a wrist injury evaluation.

The names assigned to individual ligaments have evolved based on additional information gained from anatomic dissections of their origins and insertions. Ligament names generally derive from their bony attachments, with the origin, being the more proximal or radial attachment, named first and the insertion named last. Intervening ligament attachments are named in the order of occurrence. The terms *volar* and *palmar* are synonymous, with *palmar*

being preferred; however, some conventions still require the term *volar*.

PALMAR RADIOCARPAL LIGAMENTS

The palmar radiocarpal ligaments (Fig. 1) originate from the distal palmar margin of the radius and extend to the carpus. They are stout structures and the primary stabilizers of the radiocarpal joint. Although when viewed from outside the joint they appear as a confluent sheet of capsule, these ligaments are distinguishable arthroscopically (Fig. 2). The radioscaphocapitate (RSC) ligament is the most radial of the palmar ligaments. It originates from the radial styloid and proceeds in an ulnar-oblique direction with various insertions on the waist and distal pole of the scaphoid before terminating on the neck of the capitate. It forms the radial arm, while the ulnocapitate (UC) ligament forms the ulnar arm, of what has been termed the arcuate ligament complex. The RSC ligament serves as a fulcrum around which the scaphoid flexes. An excessive radial styloidectomy may jeopardize its origin, resulting in abnormal scaphoid motion. A short oblique osteotomy with removal of only a few millimeters of articular surface preserves the radial attachment of the RSC ligament.[1] Because the standard palmar surgical approach for scaphoid fracture repair passes directly through the ligament, accurate repair and sufficient immobilization are indicated to restore its integrity. The RSC ligament should be preserved when performing a proximal row carpectomy, as it will be the only remaining palmar radiocarpal ligament.

Proceeding toward the ulna, the next ligament is the long radiolunate (LRL) ligament. The LRL ligament orig-

FIGURE 1

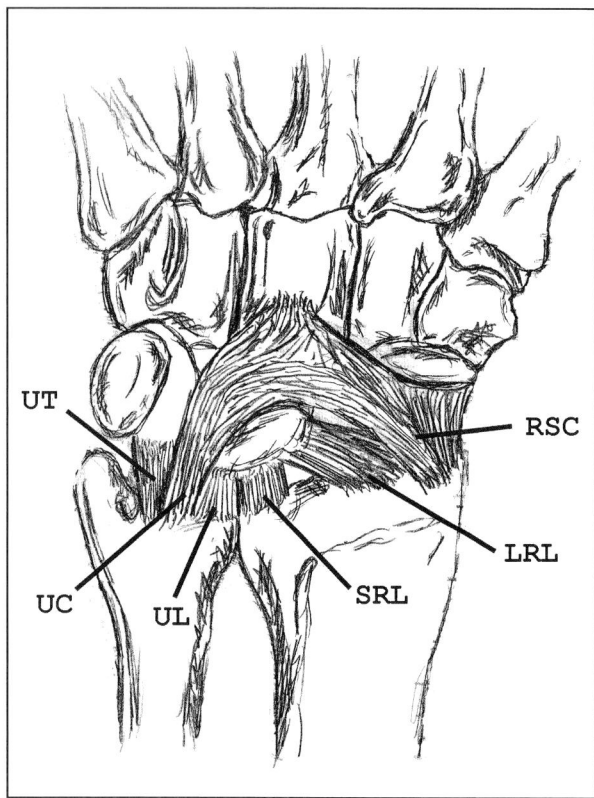

The palmar radiocarpal ligaments (palmar perspective). UT = ulnotriquetral, UC = ulnocapitate, UL = ulnolunate, SRL = short radiolunate, LRL = long radiolunate, RSC = radioscaphocapitate.

inates from the palmar rim of the scaphoid fossa and inserts onto the radial edge of the palmar horn of the lunate. The LRL was previously called the radiolunotriquetral ligament; however, because no significant fibers attach to the triquetrum, this term is less frequently used. The LRL and RSC ligaments are separated by an interligamentous sulcus, which is easily seen during arthroscopy (Fig. 3). This sulcus is the site of the palmar arthroscopic portal.

The radioscapholunate (RSL) ligament, also known as the ligament of Testut, passes along the ulnar side of the LRL ligament. It arises from the ridge between the scaphoid and lunate facets and merges into the proximal membranous portion of the scapholunate interosseous ligament (Fig. 4). Although usually called a ligament, it functions primarily as a conduit for terminal vessels and nerves from the radial artery and anterior interosseous neurovascular bundle. Studies on fetal wrists demonstrate a mesenchymal septum between the two radius facets that recedes during development, leaving the RSL ligament as a remnant.[2]

The short radiolunate (SRL) ligament is the most ulnar of the radiocarpal ligaments and is separated from the LRL ligament by the RSC ligament. It originates from the palmar rim of the lunate fossa and inserts on the proximal radial edge of the palmar horn of the lunate. The radiocarpal ligaments, in particular the SRL ligament, resist the natural tendency of the carpus to translate ulnarly down the inclined distal radius. Ulnar translation of the carpus most commonly occurs in rheumatoid arth-

FIGURE 2

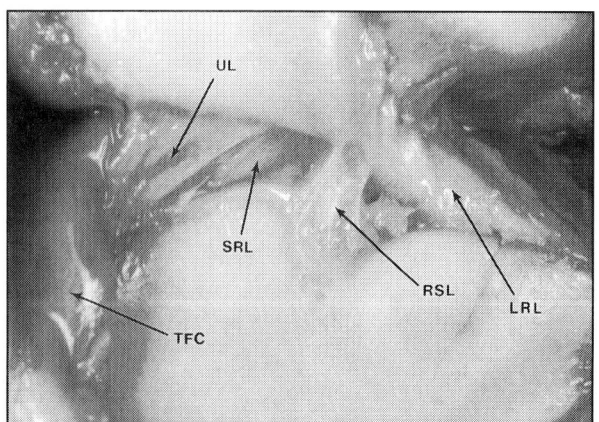

The palmar radiocarpal ligaments viewed from inside the radiocarpal joint. UL = ulnolunate, TFC = triangular fibrocartilage, SRL = short radiolunate, RSL = radioscapholunate, LRL = long radiolunate.

FIGURE 3

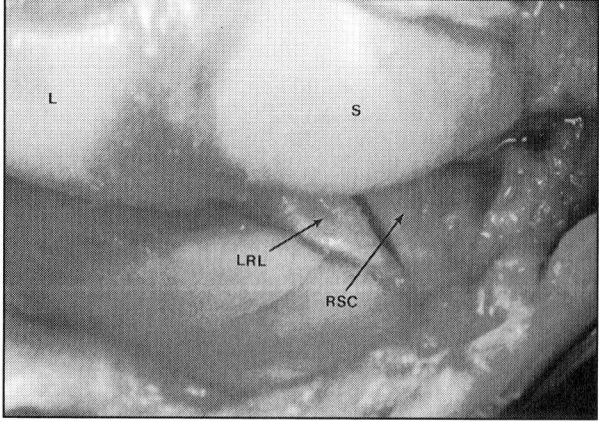

The long radiolunate (LRL) and radioscaphocapitate (RSC) ligaments arising from the palmar rim of the distal radius. Note the interligamentous sulcus between the two ligaments. L = lunate, S = scaphoid.

ritis because of gradual attenuation of the capsular ligaments. Posttraumatic ulnar translation indicates extensive injury to these ligaments and is associated with a poor prognosis.[3]

PALMAR ULNOCARPAL LIGAMENTS

Three confluent ligaments form the ulnocarpal ligament complex. The palmar ulnolunate (UL) and ulnotriquetral (UT) ligaments arise from the palmar radioulnar ligament, which is a component of the triangular fibrocartilage complex (TFCC), and insert into their respectively named carpal bones (Fig. 5). The UL ligament inserts on the ulnar portion of the palmar horn of the lunate, where it becomes confluent with the SRL ligament. The UT ligament passes to the ulnar lobe of the triquetrum, where it forms the distal portion of the extensor carpi ulnaris subsheath. The UT ligament commonly has a small distal rent that creates a communication between the radiocarpal and pisotriquetral joints. Unlike the palmar radiocarpal ligaments, the UL and UT ligaments appear as a confluent capsule when viewed arthroscopically. The UC ligament originates from the fovea of the ulnar head and the base of the ulnar styloid and lies just palmar to the UL and UT ligaments to insert on the neck of the capitate. It forms the ulnar arm of the arcuate ligament complex.

Just proximal to the apex of the arcuate ligament complex, ie, between the distal portions of the UC and RSC ligaments, the palmar wrist capsule is devoid of ligaments. This relatively weaker region of the capsule is called the space of Poirier (Fig. 6), and it is through this region that the midcarpal joint dislocates in a perilunate dislocation. Avulsion fractures of the TFCC from its ulnar attachment may cause direct injury to the UC ligament and indirect injury to the UT and UL ligaments. The palmar ulnocarpal ligaments stabilize the ulnocarpal joint, and their injury may result in a supination deformity of the carpus, often called an ulnar sag. This condition is most commonly seen in association with rheumatoid arthritis, but it can also occur following trauma.

PALMAR MIDCARPAL LIGAMENTS

The palmar midcarpal ligaments are short, stout capsular ligaments that cross a single articulation. The scaphotrapeziotrapezoid ligament passes from the palmar surface of the distal pole of the scaphoid to the palmar surface of the trapezium and trapezoid. The scaphocapitate ligament originates from the distal pole of the scaphoid and inserts on the body of the capitate. It lies parallel to the RSC ligament. The triquetrocapitate and triquetrohamate ligaments blend with the distal fibers of the UC ligament and reinforce the ulnar arm of the arcuate ligament. These ligaments are stabilizers of the scaphoid, triquetrum, and midcarpal joint.

FIGURE 4

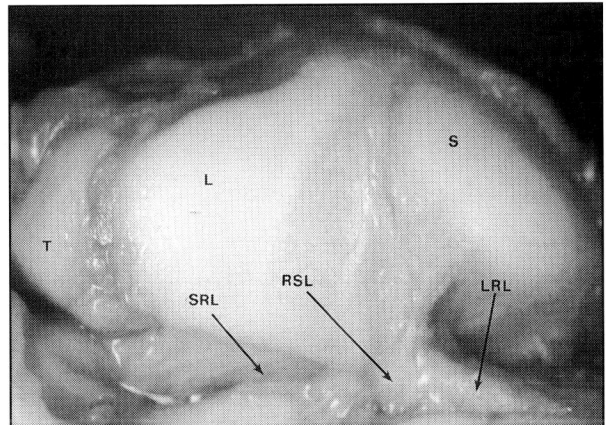

The short radiolunate, radioscapholunate, and long radiolunate ligaments. Note the insertion of the radioscapholunate ligament into the membranous component of the scapholunate interosseous ligament. T = triquetrum, L = lunate, S = scaphoid.

FIGURE 5

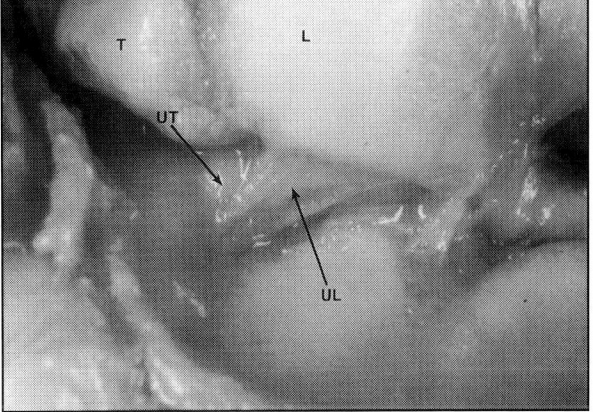

The palmar ulnocarpal ligaments viewed from inside the joint. T = triquetrum, L = lunate, UT = ulnotriquetral, UL = ulnolunate.

FIGURE 6

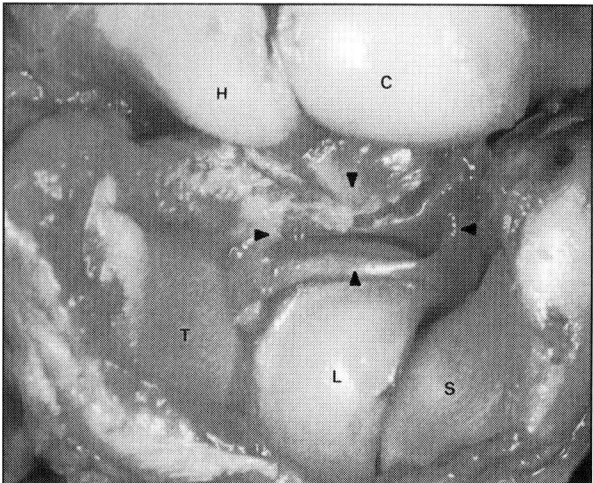

The space of Poirier (arrows). H = hamate, C = capitate, T = triquetrum, L = lunate, S = scaphoid.

DORSAL LIGAMENTS

Although the importance of the palmar wrist ligaments usually is emphasized, greater interest in and appreciation for the role of the dorsal wrist ligaments (Fig. 7) in wrist instability has developed. The dorsal radiocarpal (DRC) ligament arises from the dorsal rim of the distal radius ulnar to Lister's tubercle and inserts primarily on the dorsal aspect of the triquetrum (Fig. 8). Some of its deeper fibers also insert on the dorsal aspect of the lunate and lunotriquetral interosseous ligament. The DRC ligament controls ulnar translation of the triquetrum and stabilizes the lunate in apposition to the distal radius. The DRC ligament must be attenuated or disrupted for a static volar intercalated segment instability (VISI) to occur.[4,5]

The dorsal intercarpal (DIC) ligament originates from the dorsum of the triquetrum and inserts on the dorsal aspects of the trapezoid and the waist of the scaphoid. The DRC and DIC function together as a dorsal radioscaphoid ligament to control the scaphoid.[6] The dorsal scaphotriquetral ligament runs roughly parallel to the DIC, connecting the waist of the scaphoid to the triquetrum. It provides dorsal support for the head of the capitate. Although not shown to improve clinical results, ligament-sparing surgical approaches, which incise the capsule in line with the fibers of the DIC and DRC ligaments, have been advocated to reduce the risk of carpal instability or stiffness.[7]

FIGURE 7

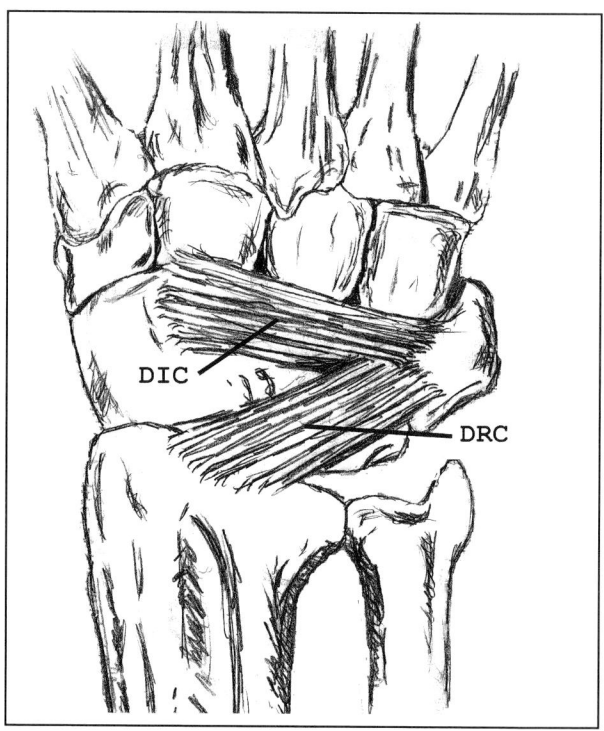

Schematic of the dorsal capsular ligaments (dorsal perspective). DIC = dorsal intercarpal, DRC = dorsal radiocarpal.

INTEROSSEOUS LIGAMENTS

Interosseous ligaments connect adjacent bones and are located entirely within the wrist capsule. The scapholunate (SL) and lunotriquetral (LT) interosseous ligaments have been the focus of considerable study because of their important roles in carpal instability.

The SL interosseous ligament is a C-shaped structure with three distinct components. The dorsal and palmar components are true ligaments. The dorsal component is more robust, with transversely oriented collagen bundles, while the palmar component is thinner, with obliquely oriented collagen bundles. The proximal component, which faces the distal radius articular surface, is avascular and consists primarily of fibrocartilage with few collagen bundles.[8]

The dorsal radiocarpal capsule typically has an attachment to the distal aspect of the dorsal component of the SL interosseous ligament. The RSL ligament blends with the juncture of the palmar and proximal components, thereby partially isolating the palmar component of the

FIGURE 8

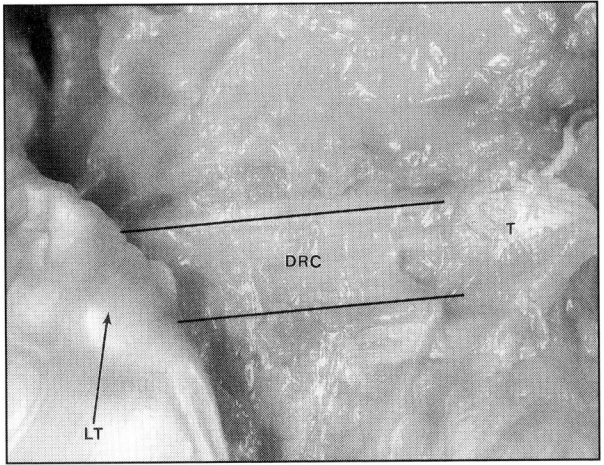

The course of the dorsal radiocarpal ligament (DRC) (indicated by horizontal lines). LT = Lister's tubercle, T = triquetrum.

radiocarpal joint. The SL interosseous ligament provides an important link between the two bones. The dorsal component is the most important for constraining scapholunate translation while the palmar component is most important for limiting rotation. Although the early in vivo effects of complete SL interosseous ligament disruption are not clear, laboratory evidence indicates that scapholunate dissociation and abnormal carpal motion result.[9]

The LT interosseous ligament is also C-shaped, with three distinct components.[10] Fibers from the ulnocarpal ligaments attach to and reinforce the palmar component. In contrast to the SL interosseous ligament, the palmar component is stronger and better resists lunotriquetral translation, while the dorsal component better resists lunotriquetral rotation. Several laboratory studies have sought to determine the role of the LT interosseous ligament in ulnar-sided wrist instability.[4,5,11] Its complete disruption is necessary but not sufficient for a static VISI deformity to develop; injury to additional ligaments is also required.

Interosseous ligaments are present within the distal carpal row between the trapezium and trapezoid, trapezium and capitate, and capitate and hamate. These ligaments are short and stout, with dorsal and palmar components. In addition, there are intra-articular ligaments connecting the trapezium and the capitate, and the capitate and the hamate. The combination of highly congruous articular surfaces and this complex of ligaments creates a tight bond among the bones of the distal carpal row, resulting in a single functioning skeletal unit.

SUMMARY

The complex nature of the articulations, ligaments, and motions of the wrist has generated tremendous interest, debate, and frustration among clinical and laboratory investigators. The anatomy of the wrist ligaments described in this chapter is the product of numerous investigators over several decades. Despite this enormous effort, our current understanding of ligament function remains preliminary. While certain ligaments appear to be essential for normal function, no ligament acts in isolation to control motion or to prevent carpal malalignment. In vivo study using new technologies likely offers the next step in defining the function of wrist ligaments.

REFERENCES

1. Siegel DB, Gelberman RH: Radial styloidectomy: An anatomical study with special reference to radiocarpal intracapsular ligamentous morphology. *J Hand Surg Am* 1991;16:40-44.
2. Berger RA, Kauer JM, Landsmeer JM: Radioscapholunate ligament: A gross anatomic and histologic study of fetal and adult wrists. *J Hand Surg Am* 1991;16:350-355.
3. Viegas SF, Patterson RM, Ward K: Extrinsic wrist ligaments in the pathomechanics of ulnar translation instability. *J Hand Surg Am* 1995;20:312-318.
4. Viegas SF, Patterson RM, Peterson PD, et al: Ulnar-sided perilunate instability: An anatomic and biomechanic study. *J Hand Surg Am* 1990;15:268-278.
5. Horii E, Garcia-Elias M, An KN, et al: A kinematic study of luno-triquetral dissociations. *J Hand Surg Am* 1991;16: 355-362.
6. Viegas SF, Yamaguchi S, Boyd NL, Patterson RM: The dorsal ligaments of the wrist: Anatomy, mechanical properties, and function. *J Hand Surg Am* 1999;24:456-468.
7. Berger RA, Bishop AT, Bettinger PC: New dorsal capsulotomy for the surgical exposure of the wrist. *Ann Plast Surg* 1995;35:54-59.
8. Berger RA: The gross and histologic anatomy of the scapholunate interosseous ligament. *J Hand Surg Am* 1996;21:170-178.
9. Ruby LK, An KN, Linscheid RL, Cooney WP III, Chao EY: The effect of scapholunate ligament section on scapholunate motion. *J Hand Surg Am* 1987;12:767-771.
10. Ritt MJ, Bishop AT, Berger RA, Linscheid RL, Berglund LJ, An KN: Lunotriquetral ligament properties: A comparison of three anatomic subregions. *J Hand Surg Am* 1998;23:425-431.
11. Trumble TE, Bour CJ, Smith RJ, Glisson RR: Kinematics of the ulnar carpus related to the volar intercalated segment instability pattern. *J Hand Surg Am* 1990;15: 384-392.

CHAPTER 2

BIOMECHANICAL STUDIES OF WRIST LIGAMENT INJURIES

ALEXANDER Y. SHIN, MD
PETER M. MURRAY, MD

The mechanics and function of the human wrist joint are unique. Unlike the elbow or shoulder, which have simple mechanical equivalents (hinged joint and ball-and-socket joint, respectively), the wrist has no simple equivalent. The wrist is a diarthrodial joint composed of two rows of carpal bones. The proximal row articulates with the distal articular surface of the radius, which consists of the scaphoid fossa and the lunate fossa. The distal surfaces of the scaphoid, lunate, and triquetrum accept the contours of the distal carpal row, comprised of the trapezium, trapezoid, capitate, and hamate. The proximal articulation of the wrist is the radiocarpal joint; the distal articulation is the midcarpal joint. The 15 osseous elements of the human carpus, therefore, form six major articulations (radiocarpal, midcarpal, pisotriquetral, trapeziometacarpal, common carpometacarpal, and the distal radioulnar joints), each with multiple subarticulations. The extrinsic and intrinsic ligaments, described in chapter 1, connect and stabilize the osseous elements, while the flexor and extensor tendons cross over the carpus, influencing the wrist through the transmission of force. The intrinsic ligaments are the biomechanical glue that holds the bones of the proximal and distal carpal rows together. The pisiform articulates with the palmar aspect of the triquetrum and is encapsulated by a large synovial cavity. In approximately 30% of the population, the pisotriquetral joint communicates directly with the radiocarpal joint.[1]

Each of the carpal bones is unique in its mechanics and possesses a unique center of rotation. The overall motion in the wrist is, in essence, the sum of the carpal bones moving on each other, influenced by their articulations, ligamentous attachments, and indirect actions of adjacent tendons. These interactions of the carpal bones have been compared to the mechanism of a Rubik's cube, where motion in one segment directly affects the position of the other segments.[2]

A clear understanding of the normal biomechanics of the wrist contributes to a better understanding of the mechanisms of wrist injuries, which helps to determine appropriate treatment. The purpose of this chapter is to describe the following biomechanical concepts and their clinical application: normal carpal mechanics, the classification of carpal instabilities, the material properties of wrist ligaments, and the mechanisms of carpal injuries.

NORMAL CARPAL MECHANICS

Carpal instabilities result from fracture or from alterations in individual carpal ligaments. Insight into normal carpal mechanics can allow clearer and more accurate evaluations of the mechanics of carpal derangement.[3-7] Destot[8] and Navarro[9] conducted pioneering work in this area in the early 1900s, but it was largely neglected until Gilford and associates[10] introduced the concept of carpal instability associated with scaphoid fractures in 1943. Further contributions by Fisk,[11] Linscheid and associates,[12-14] Mayfield and associates,[15-17] Taleisnik,[18-20] Lichtman and associates,[21-23] and Watson and associates[24-26] have provided tremendous insight into the understanding of carpal mechanics and wrist injury.

With the use of implanted metal markers in the carpal bones of cadaveric wrists, Andrews and Youm,[27] Youm and Yoon,[28] McMurtry and associates,[29] and Youm and associates[30] demonstrated the biaxial nature of the carpus, establishing the principle that the wrist maintains a constant carpal height ratio during wrist radial and ulnar deviation. This ratio was defined as the distance from the base

FIGURE 1

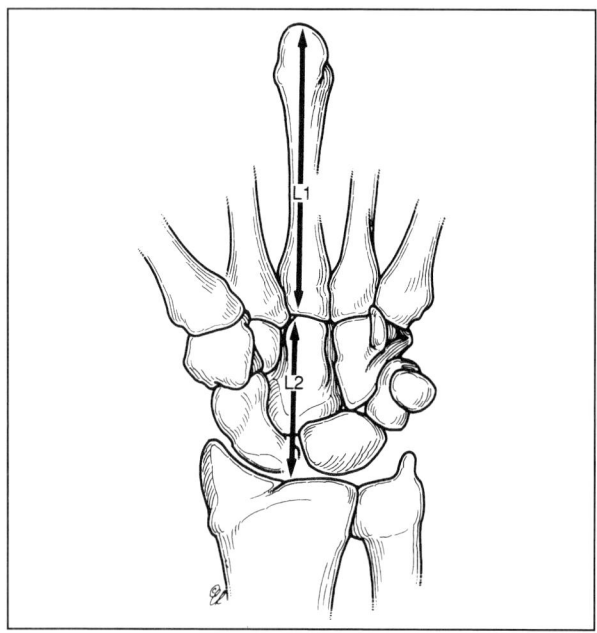

The carpal height ratio is calculated by dividing the carpal height (L2) by the length of the third metacarpal (L1). The normal ratio, 0.54 ± 0.03, is maintained in all positions of wrist motion. (Reproduced with permission from Garcia-Elias M: Carpal instabilities and dislocations, in Green DP, Hotchkiss RN, Pederson WC (eds): *Green's Operative Hand Surgery*, ed 4. New York, NY, Churchill Livingstone, 1999, pp 865-928.)

of the third metacarpal to the distal subchondral plate of the radius, divided by the length of the third metacarpal. This normal carpal height ratio is 0.54 ± 0.03 (Fig. 1).

The concept that carpal bones are grouped into rigid columns, as suggested by Navarro,[9] was challenged by Berger and associates,[4] who performed the first quantitative analysis of the relative motion between carpal bones. Using sound sources implanted in carpal bones and a three-dimensional sonic digitizer, the authors recorded the magnitudes and direction of rotation for each carpal bone. Small but significant independent motion of each of the carpal bones was found, in contradiction to Navarro's columnar theory of wrist motion.

Accurate radiographic stereophotogrammetric measurement systems also have been used to evaluate carpal bone motion;[31,32] these studies have confirmed that significant motion does exist between carpal bones during wrist motion. The proximal carpal row is an intercalated segment with no tendon attachments. All the tendons that influence wrist motion insert distally, either onto the base of the metacarpals (flexor carpi radialis, extensor carpi radialis longus, extensor carpi radialis brevis, extensor carpi ulnaris) or onto the pisiform (flexor carpi ulnaris). The latter has distal ligamentous attachments to the hook of the hamate and the base of the fourth and fifth metacarpals. Because of this arrangement, wrist motion in any plane must be initiated at the distal carpal row. Proximal carpal row motion commences only when the extrinsic ligaments crossing the midcarpal joint become taut and the compressive forces exerted on the proximal carpal row reach a threshold that exceeds the frictional forces of the intervening articular segments and the resistance of antagonistic muscular forces.

Although some motion occurs between the individual bones of the distal carpal row, these bones, with the index and middle metacarpals, function as a single unit.[4,33,34] Because of the articular geometry of the midcarpal joint, unconstrained wrist motion produces multiplanar motion of the distal carpal row. During flexion of the wrist, the distal carpal row flexes and deviates slightly ulnarly. With extension, the distal carpal row extends and deviates radially. With radial deviation, the distal carpal row deviates radially, extends, and supinates. With ulnar deviation of the wrist, the distal carpal row deviates ulnarly, flexes, and pronates.[35] Thus, the relationship between the distal carpal row and the index and middle metacarpals is maintained throughout all directions and magnitudes of motion.[36] The bones of the proximal carpal row are less tightly bound to one another than are those of the distal carpal row.[4,5,31,37] The relative motion of the scaphoid, lunate, and triquetrum differs considerably.[2,4,6,31,32,38-41] Because of the significant motion between the bones that comprise it, the proximal carpal row cannot be considered a single functional unit.

In the normal wrist, a balanced synchrony is maintained between the proximal and distal carpal rows.[36,42] Descriptions of motion in the flexion-extension plane and in radial and ulnar deviation follow (Fig. 2).

When motion occurs in the flexion-extension plane, there is coordinated motion between the distal and proximal carpal rows. As the distal carpal row flexes, the proximal carpal row also flexes. Similarly, when the distal carpal row extends, the proximal carpal row extends. The relative contribution of flexion and extension of each of the carpal rows depends on the frame of reference evaluated. If the central portion of the carpus (capitate-lunate-radius linkage) is considered, radiocarpal and midcarpal motion is equally divided in one third of wrists; the remaining two thirds experience approximately 60% of flexion at the midcarpal joint and 66% of extension at the radiocarpal joint.[5,32,43] However, when the frame of reference is

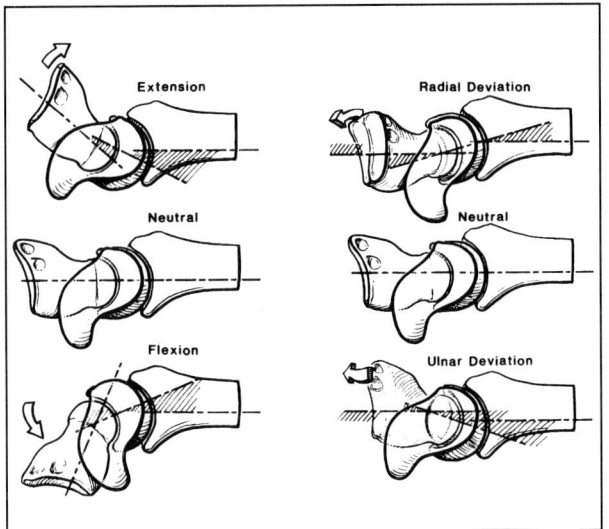

In flexion and extension, the proximal and distal carpal rows move synergistically. However, radial-ulnar deviation involves a reciprocal flexion and extension of the proximal carpal row. In radial deviation of the wrist, the distal carpal bones undergo radial deviation and extension while the proximal carpal row flexes and translates ulnarly. In ulnar deviation of the wrist, the distal carpal bones undergo ulnar deviation and flexion while the proximal carpal row extends and translates radially. (Reproduced with permission from Amadio PC: Carpal kinematics and instability: A clinical and anatomic primer. *Clin Anat* 1991;4:1-12.)

changed to the lateral portion of the carpus (radius-scaphoid-trapezium linkage), nearly two thirds of the global arc of motion occurs at the radioscaphoid joint.[3,5,40]

Radial or ulnar deviation involves a complex reciprocating motion of the proximal and distal carpal rows. With radial deviation, the distal carpal row inclines radially and extends and supinates. The proximal carpal bones principally flex and translate ulnarly. With ulnar deviation, the opposite occurs. The distal carpal row inclines ulnarly and flexes and pronates, whereas the proximal carpal bones extend and translate radially.[6,40,44] These complex motions are required to maintain the carpal congruency and spatial consistency in all wrist positions.[5,45,46]

CLASSIFICATION OF CARPAL INSTABILITIES

Descriptions of instability of the carpal bones first appeared shortly after the advent of radiographs.[8-11,47] However, the biomechanical implications of these descriptions were poorly understood until 1972, when Linscheid

and associates[12] described carpal instability based on the position of the lunate, introducing the terms dorsal intercalated segmental instability (DISI) and volar intercalated segmental instability (VISI). In 1980, Mayfield and associates[16] introduced the concept of perilunate instability, demonstrating a progressive injury centered about the lunate and initiated on the radial aspect of the wrist. Two years later, Reagan and associates[48] improved the understanding of ulnar-sided wrist instability in their description of lunotriquetral instability. During the 1980s the concept of instability of the entire proximal carpal row was further advanced and variously termed triquetrohamate, midcarpal, and capitolunate instability.[18,19,21-23,49,50] Garcia-Elias and associates[51-53] defined axial carpal disruptions in 1989, and in 1993, Watson and associates[24] introduced the concept of dynamic carpal instability. In an attempt to unify wrist instability theory, several authors devised a more refined and complete classification[36,42,54] (Table 1).

Dissociative Instability

Carpal instability, dissociative (CID), occurs between or through the bones of the same carpal row, causing dissociation within the row. CID can occur in either the proximal or distal carpal row, secondary to a ligament injury or fracture. Of proximal row dissociative instability patterns, scapholunate dissociation is the most recognized. Unstable fractures of the scaphoid, lunate, or triquetrum can also result in this pattern. For the dissociative pattern to occur, the injury must completely disrupt the scapholunate interosseous ligament (SLIL).

Nondissociative Instability

Carpal instability, nondissociative (CIND), includes instability patterns that occur between a carpal row and the adjacent transverse osseous structures. In these patterns, there is no dissociation within the carpal rows (ie, competent interosseous ligaments). These instability patterns include midcarpal instabilities,[21-23] ulnar translocations,[55,56] capitolunate instability patterns,[50,57] and proximal carpal row instabilities.[49] CIND can occur secondary to fractures, disruption or laxity of extrinsic ligaments, or both.

Combined or Complex Instability

Carpal instability, combined or complex (CIC), is a combination of two or more specific CID or CIND patterns. Examples of the complex instability include perilunate dislocations, radiocarpal instability with axial instability, and scapholunate dissociation with ulnar translocation.

TABLE 1

Mayo Clinic Classification of Carpal Instability

Type of Instability	Radiographic Pattern	Type of Instability	Radiographic Pattern
Carpal Instability, Dissociative (CID)		Combined radiocarpal-midcarpal CIND	
Proximal carpal row CID		CLIP	VISI, DISI, alternating
Unstable scaphoid fracture	DISI		
Scapholunate dissociation	DISI	Disruption of central and radial	UT±VISI
Lunotriquetral dissociation	±VISI	ligaments	or DISI
Distal carpal row CID			
Axial-radial disruption	RT, PT	Carpal Instability, Combined or Complex (CIC)	
Axial-ulnar disruption	UT, PT	Perilunate with radiocarpal instability	DISI & UT
Combined axial-radial-ulnar		Perilunate with axial instability	AxUI & UT
Combined proximal and distal CID		Radiocarpal with axial instability	AxRI & UT
		Scapholunate dissociation with	DISI & UT
		ulnar translocation	
Carpal Instability, Nondissociative (CIND)			
Radiocarpal CIND		Carpal Instability, Adaptive	
Palmar ligament rupture	DISI, UT	Malposition of the carpus with	DISI or DT
	UT, PT	distal radius malunion	
	VISI, DT	Malposition of the carpus with	DISI
Dorsal ligament rupture	VISI, DT	scaphoid nonunion	
Midcarpal CIND		Malposition of the carpus with	DISI or VISI
Ulnar MCI from palmar ligament	VISI	lunate malunion	
damage		Malposition of the carpus with	UT, DISI, PT
Radial MCI from palmar ligament	VISI	Madelung's deformity	
damage			
Combined ulnar and radial	VISI		
MCI from dorsal ligament damage	DISI		

AR = axial-radial; AU = axial-ulnar; AxRI = axial-radial instability; AxUI = axial-ulnar instability; CLIP = capitolunate instability pattern; DISI = dorsal intercalated segmental instability; VISI = volar intercalated segmental instability; DT = dorsal translation; MCI = midcarpal instability; PT = proximal translation; RT = radial translation; UT = ulnar translation.

(Reproduced with permission from Dobyns JH, Cooney WP: Classification of carpal instability, in Cooney WP, Linscheid RL, Dobyns JH (eds): *The Wrist: Diagnosis and Operative Treatment*. St Louis, MO, Mosby, 1998.)

Adaptive Instability

Adaptive carpal instability results from the repositioning of the carpus in response to a change in the bony architecture.[19,20,55] One of the more common etiologies of an adaptive instability is the dorsally angulated distal radius malunion, which results in a compensatory DISI of the carpus. Other types of adaptive instability include those secondary to scaphoid nonunions, lunate malunions, or Madelung's deformity.

WRIST LIGAMENT PROPERTIES AND BIOMECHANICS

The human wrist joint articulates in flexion and extension as well as in radial and ulnar deviation. Pronation and supination of the forearm also position the carpus. Intracarpal supination and pronation as well as radiocarpal translation further modify these active wrist movements. As previously outlined, the motion of the carpus is synchronous between the radiocarpal and the midcarpal joints. The proximal carpal row is an intercalated segment devoid of tendon insertion and directly influenced by the motion of the distal carpal row.[12] In describing this carpal motion, Linscheid and associates[12] likened the movements of the proximal and distal carpal rows to a "slider-crank," a three-bar linkage mechanism with the scaphoid representing the crank. The scaphoid, because of its position, has potential energy for flexion, while the triquetrum, because of its helicoid articulation with the hamate, has potential energy for extension.[58] This potential energy created in the proximal carpal row is facilitated by the SLIL, which stabilizes the scaphoid and the lunate, and the lunotriquetral interosseous ligament (LTIL), which stabilizes the lunate and the triquetrum. The result is a dynamic, balanced lunate within the proximal carpal row. During radial deviation, the proximal carpal row translates toward the ulna, while the distal carpal row inclines toward the radius. Additionally, the scaphoid must flex to avoid impinging on the radial styloid, and the entire proximal row is pulled into flexion as long as there is integrity of the SLIL. In ulnar deviation of the carpus, the triquetrum is forced into extension by its helicoid articulation with the hamate. This pushes the remainder of the proximal carpal row into extension by virtue of the force transmission through the LTIL.[58] In contrast, the distal carpal row has negligible intracarpal motion, being generally bound together by very short, stout ligaments with broad insertions.[34]

Ligaments, in general, are composed of 90% type I collagen and 10% type III collagen.[59] Because of their composition, wrist ligaments function primarily as viscoelastic structures.[60] Knowing the absolute strength of the ligaments helps us to understand their importance in the kinematics of the wrist. The extrinsic ligaments of the wrist, such as the radioscaphocapitate (RSC) ligament and the long radiolunate (LRL) ligament, have viscoelastic properties similar to other human ligaments, with failure force in tension of approximately 100 to 200 N.[61,62] Values of strain at ultimate stress for the extrinsic wrist ligaments range from 20% to 125%.[61,62] In contrast, the radioscapholunate ligament, once thought to have mechanical properties similar to the other extrinsic ligaments, is now known to possess substantial vascular tissue,[63] with elastin contributing to its elastic behavior. Furthermore, the structure is relatively weak and elastic, with a tensile strength of 50 N and 150% strain at maximum stress.[62] Although it has been suggested that the flexor retinaculum functions as a carpal stabilizer, in one biomechanical analysis it was shown that sectioning the flexor retinaculum has little effect on the transverse stability of the carpus.[52,53] In general, the extrinsic ligaments of the wrist are weaker and stiffer than the intrinsic ligaments.[61,62,64]

The SLIL has been found to be particularly strong, failing at approximately 300 N of longitudinal load.[61,62] The SLIL is composed of three distinct portions: proximal, dorsal, and palmar.[65] The dorsal portion of the SLIL is the strongest, followed by the palmar portion; the proximal or membranous portion provides very little stability to the scapholunate articulation.[66] Using a cadaveric model, significantly different translation and rotation of the scapholunate interval can be demonstrated with isolated sectioning of the dorsal portion of the SLIL. In contrast, sectioning of the proximal and palmar portions of the SLIL, using the same cadaveric model, has not shown significant changes in translation or rotation.[66] The SLIL possesses failure strength in tension, which, in one study, is nearly double that of the RSC ligament.[61] The LTIL and the capitohamate interosseous ligament (CHIL) have been shown to possess strength and stiffness characteristics similar to those of the dorsal portion of the SLIL (the LTIL fails at approximately 350 N; the CHIL has an ultimate strength of approximately 250 N).[60,62] The relative contribution of the CHIL to distal carpal row stability has been illustrated using a mathematical model. This mathematical model simulated sectioning of the palmar portion of the CHIL, which produced significant destabilization of the distal carpal row, implicating this structure as the primary stabilizer of the distal carpal row.[52,53] In both the intrinsic and the extrinsic wrist ligaments, a significantly greater failure force in tension and strain at ultimate stress can be demonstrated with higher rates of elongation.[62]

The relatively greater strength and viscoelastic nature of the interosseous ligaments reflect their functional characteristics and anatomy. The complex, intercalated movements of the proximal carpal row are facilitated by the interosseous ligaments, which are strong and particularly accommodating to shear stress. The extrinsic wrist ligaments, by contrast, are much weaker and stiffer because there is little need for these structures to have dynamic capabilities.

MECHANISMS OF CARPAL DISRUPTIONS

Radial-Sided Carpal Instabilities

Collectively, perilunate and lunate dislocations, as well as scapholunate dissociations, have been referred to as radial-

TABLE 2

Radiographic and Anatomic Findings in the Four Stages of Perilunate Instability[16]

	Stage I	Stage II	Stage III	Stage IV
Radiographic manifestations	Scaphoid rotation Scapholunate dissociation	Dislocated capitate	Malrotated triquetrum and scaphoid Lunotriquetral dissociation Dislocated triquetrum Palmar triquetral fracture	Lunate dislocation
Joint(s) disrupted	Scapholunate	Scapholunate Capitolunate	Scapholunate Capitolunate Lunotriquetral	Scapholunate Capitolunate Lunotriquetral Radiolunate
Ligaments torn or attenuated	Radioscaphoid Scapholunate Radiocapitate	Radioscaphoid Scapholunate Radiocapitate Radial collateral	Radioscaphoid Scapholunate Radiocapitate Radial collateral Radiocapitate Palmar radiotriquetral at triquetrolunate joint Ulnotriquetral with or without dorsal radiocarpal	Radioscaphoid Scapholunate Radiocapitate Radial collateral Radiocapitate Palmar radiotriquetral at triquetrolunate joint Ulnotriquetral with or without dorsal radiocarpal

Reproduced with permission from Mayfield JK, Johnson RP, Kilcoyne RK: Carpal dislocations: Pathomechanics and progressive perilunar instability. *J Hand Surg Am* 1980;5:226-241.

sided perilunate instabilities because the mechanism of injury is presumed to be initiated on the radial side of the wrist. Prior to 1980, most authors agreed that perilunate injuries occurred with forced extension and that they involved dislocation of the capitate from the lunate and separation of the scaphoid from the lunate by either a fracture or a ligament disruption. The mechanism of perilunate dislocations remained poorly understood, however, until Mayfield and associates[16,17] introduced the concept of progressive perilunate instability. In their study, the authors loaded cadaveric wrists in extension, ulnar deviation, and intercarpal supination to simulate the perilunate and the lunate dislocations. Radial-sided carpal

instabilities, which occur following injury caused by a compressive force across a hyperdorsiflexed wrist, are a spectrum of injuries with a common mechanism: hyperdorsiflexion of the wrist, forearm pronation, ulnar deviation of the hand, and axial loading of the wrist through the radial palm and thenar eminence, as previously mentioned.[16,17] Through radiographic evaluation and dissection of the specimens, four distinct patterns of injury emerged (Table 2), collectively termed "progressive perilunate instability." The authors deemed that this progression occurred in four stages. In stage I, disruption of the SLIL and RSC occurs. In stage II, the capitate and scaphoid separate from the lunate and the triquetrum. In stage III,

FIGURE 3

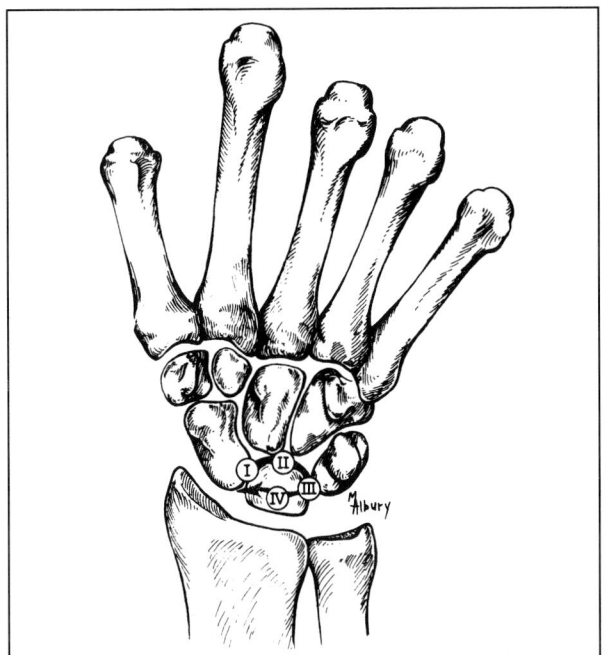

The stages of progressive perilunate instability include stage I (scapholunate dissociation), stage II (capitolunate dissociation), stage III (lunotriquetral dissociation), and stage IV (complete lunate dislocation). (Reproduced with permission from Mayfield JK: Mechanism of carpal injuries. *Clin Orthop* 1980;149:45-54.)

FIGURE 4

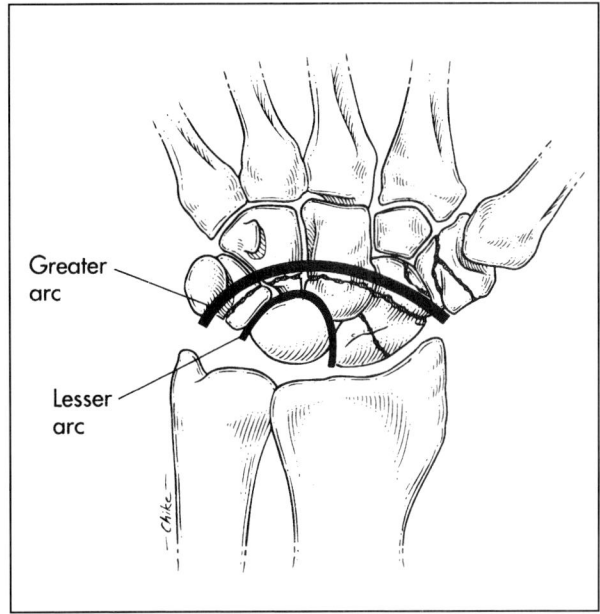

Palmar view of a right hand showing the pathways of ligamentous and bone injury about the wrist. The lesser arc injuries represent the ligamentous disruptions described by Mayfield and associates. Greater arc injuries are those that occur through the carpal bones. (Reproduced with permission from Kozin SH, Murphy MS, Cooney WP: Perilunate dislocations, in Cooney WP, Linscheid RL, Dobyns JH (eds): *The Wrist: Diagnosis and Operative Treatment.* St Louis, MO, Mosby, 1998.)

the injury continues ulnarly and separates the triquetrum from the lunate. At stage III, the carpus is completely separated from the lunate, resulting in a perilunate dislocation. Finally, in stage IV, there is a complete lunate dislocation (Fig. 3). The perilunate and the lunate dislocations may occur in a dorsal or palmar direction.

Fractures associated with perilunate dislocations are given the prefix *trans-* and represent "greater arc" injuries. The term "lesser arc" injury is reserved for the pure perilunate dislocation, without fractures. The pure greater arc injury propagates in a transscaphoid, transcapitate, and transtriquetral fashion (Fig. 4). Typically, these injuries occur secondary to high-energy trauma, and the position of the wrist at the time of injury will determine the fracture-dislocation pattern. It has been postulated that greater arc injuries result from high-energy three-dimensional loading of the wrist with axial and torsional forces applied to any combination of hyperextension, hyperflexion, and radial or ulnar deviation.[67-69] Ultimately, it is the type of loading (slow versus fast), the magnitude and direction of the forces applied, and the individual bio-

mechanical properties of the ligaments and bone that determine the fracture-dislocation pattern.

Ulnar-Sided Wrist Ligament Injuries

Less well recognized, less understood, and much less common are perilunate wrist injuries initiated on the ulnar side of the wrist. LTIL injuries also occur along a spectrum, beginning with simple ligament tears[48] and progressing to static VISI.[39,48] Alterations in lunotriquetral articulation positioning and mobility during physiologic loading have been demonstrated after LTIL sectioning.[6] Static collapse or dissociation of the lunotriquetral articulation, however, has not been demonstrated after simple sectioning of the LTIL.[39] Further sectioning of the dorsal radiotriquetral and the dorsal scaphotriquetral ligaments is required to create the static VISI position deformity.[6,39,70]

Palmar triquetral avulsion fractures involve injury of the ulnotriquetral and ulnolunate (ulnar leash) ligament complex.[71] The observation of this injury prompted a biomechanical cadaveric study that demonstrated a progres-

FIGURE 5

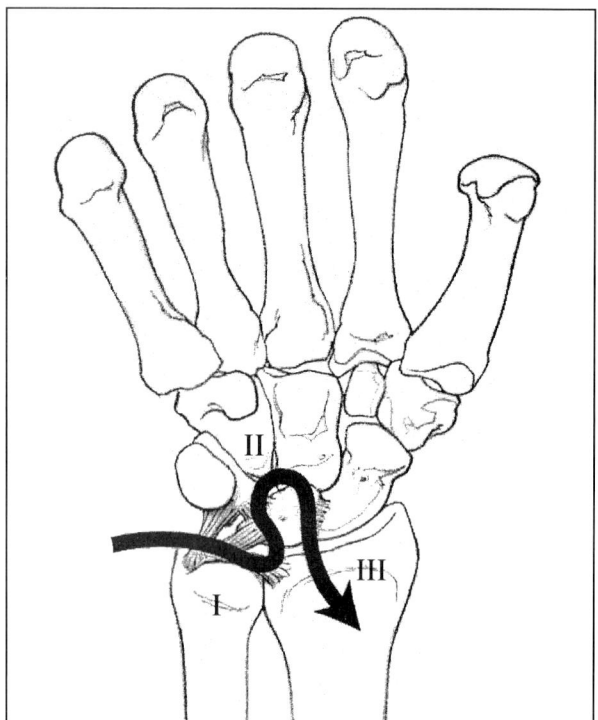

The mechanism of ulnar-sided perilunate instability. Stage I: Disruption of the ulnolunate and ulnotriquetral (ulnar leash) ligament complex. Stage II: Lunotriquetral interosseous ligament disruption. Stage III: Progression of the injury through the midcarpal joint and disruption of the scapholunate interosseous ligament.

FIGURE 6

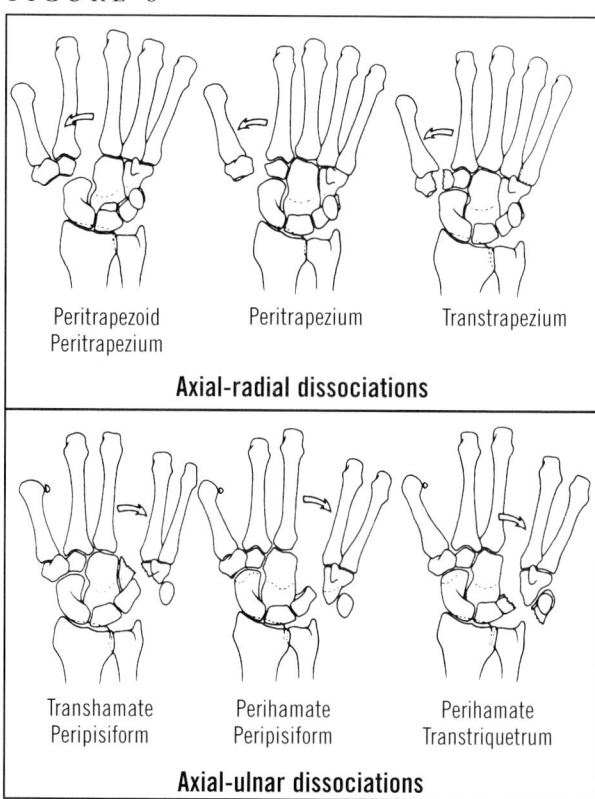

The classification of axial carpal dissociations includes the axial-radial, axial-ulnar, and axial-radial-ulnar dissociations. In axial-radial dissociations, an unstable segment displaces radially. In axial-ulnar dissociations, the displacement is toward the ulna. In the combined axial-radial-ulnar dissociation, two segments are displaced, one radially and the other ulnarly. (Reproduced with permission from Garcia-Elias M, Dobyns JH, Cooney WP III, Linscheid RL: Traumatic axial dislocations of the carpus. *J Hand Surg Am* 1989;14:446-457.)

sive perilunate injury pattern, initiated on the ulnar side of the wrist.[72] The authors demonstrated progressive perilunate disruption with axial loading of forearm specimens positioned in wrist hyperextension and radial deviation (Fig. 5), which they described as a three-stage injury mechanism: Stage I is a tear of the LTIL; stage II is disruption of the palmar ulnar leash complex as well as the dorsal radiotriquetral and the dorsal scaphotriquetral ligaments; and stage III is a tear of the SLIL with the development of a perilunate dislocation in some specimens.[72] The authors conclude that this "reverse" perilunate injury may occur also by falling on an outstretched, hyperextended wrist.

Axial Carpal Instability

Axial disruptions of the wrist are rare and usually occur secondary to high-energy crush or blast injuries.[51] The term *axial-loading dislocation* describes a derangement of the carpus that is oriented parallel to the long axis

of the forearm.[73] Other terms that describe similar disruptions of the distal carpal row include longitudinal disruption,[74] capitohamate diastasis,[75] carpal arch disruption,[76] and columnar dislocations.[51]

In axial carpal disruption, the normal convexity of the metacarpal arch is flattened, rotational deformities of the fingers occur, and the carpometacarpal junction is widened.[76,77] The spectrum of axial carpal instability ranges from acute, gross traumatic fracture-dislocations with severe soft-tissue trauma to chronic dynamic instability between the axial components of the carpus.[78]

Garcia-Elias and associates[51] classified axial dislocations of the carpus into three groups according to the direction of instability: axial-ulnar disruptions, axial-radial disruptions, and combined axial-radial-ulnar disruptions.

FIGURE 7

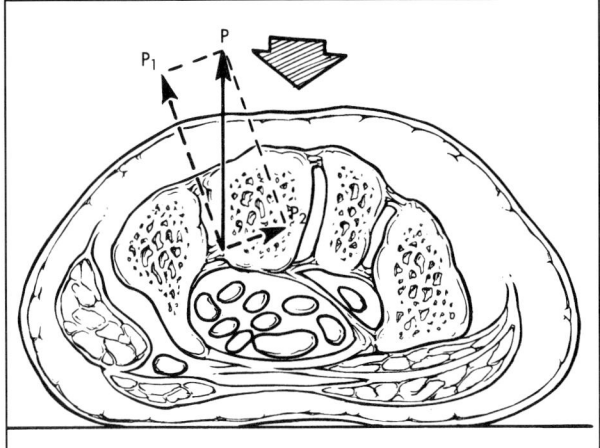

The transverse carpal arch under a dorsopalmar compression. The reaction forces of the joint are made up of two vectors, P1 and P2: P1 (shear) is tangential to the articular surface, and P2 (compression) is perpendicular to P1. If the obliqueness of the joint is great, then the shear forces will overcome the compressive forces, and dislocation is likely to occur. However, if compressive forces are higher than the shear forces, the bones will probably fracture. (Reproduced with permission from Garcia-Elias M, Cooney WP: Axial dislocations and fracture dislocations, in Cooney WP, Linscheid RL, Dobyns JH (eds): *The Wrist: Diagnosis and Operative Treatment.* St Louis, MO, Mosby, 1998.)

In axial-ulnar disruptions, the carpus splits into two columns, with the radial column stable with respect to the radius and the ulnar column (with the metacarpals) displaced ulnarly and proximally. In axial-radial disruptions, the ulnar column is stable with respect to the radius, and the radial column (including the metacarpals) displaces proximally and radially. A combination of ulnar and radial displacement of the columns is classified as an axial-radial-ulnar disruption (Fig. 6).

The typical mechanism of injury of axial carpal disruptions is a crush (eg, from a molding press, roller press, or wringer machine), twisting, or blast injury.[51,73,76] Most reported axial carpal dislocations have been industrial injuries.[51,77,79-81] The most common mechanism of injury is a dorsopalmar compression or crush of the wrist. With sufficient dorsopalmar force applied to the entire wrist, the carpal bones will either dislocate or sustain sagittally oriented fractures. The more closely parallel the intercarpal joint is to the direction of force, the greater the likelihood for dislocation. With increasing obliquity of the intercarpal joint to the direction of force, the greater the likelihood for fracture in the sagittal plane (Fig. 7).

CLINICAL APPLICATION OF EXPERIMENTAL DATA

Biomechanical studies of the wrist conducted in the 20th century have contributed greatly to the understanding of carpal mechanics and wrist instabilities. The unique nature of the ligamentous scaffolding of the human carpus and the intricacy of carpal articulations are now well recognized. The differential material properties of the extrinsic and intrinsic carpal ligaments are enhanced by the availability of a complicated reciprocating and synchronous motion. This understanding of the important relationships between the unique nature of carpal ligaments and the carpal articular surfaces has facilitated treatment that restores as nearly as possible the integrity of these structures. More than any other wrist biomechanics theory, the concept of the intercalated segment advanced the understanding of carpal kinematics. Building on this concept, the instability patterns of DISI and VISI were described and later included in a more complete classification system on which treatment algorithms have been based. Additionally, cadaveric loading studies have elucidated the progression of ligamentous insults about the wrist. These studies provide some understanding of the extent of major carpal ligamentous disruption, enabling the clinician to identify appropriate treatment alternatives.

In acute SLIL disruptions, ligament repair is generally favored over more restrictive procedures such as limited carpal arthrodesis or pancarpal arthrodesis.[12,82] Furthermore, there is compelling evidence that reconstruction of the native SLIL with anatomic restoration of the radiocarpal and midcarpal articular surfaces provides the best treatment for the perilunate dislocation.[83,84] Our enhanced knowledge of the material properties of the individual carpal ligaments has prompted the development of technically specific repair techniques. For example, studies have established that the SLIL is composed of three distinct regions and that the dorsal portion retains the greatest relative failure strength in tension; therefore, repair and reconstructive efforts have been limited to that portion of the ligament.

SUMMARY

The human carpus is a complex diarthrodial joint with 15 osseous elements and six articulations. A complex arrangement of extrinsic and intrinsic ligaments stabilizes the wrist while allowing motion in multiple planes. The extrinsic, or capsular, ligaments are weaker and stiffer than the intrinsic, or interosseous, ligaments. The viscoelastic nature of the intrinsic ligaments allows relative motion between the bones of the proximal carpal row while maintaining stability. The lunate is the intercalated segment of the proximal row, and the proximal carpal row is the intercalated segment of the carpus, each influenced by forces acting around it. Radial deviation requires flexion of the proximal carpal row, while ulnar deviation requires proximal carpal row extension because of the helicoid articulation of the triquetral-hamate articulation. The normal wrist is, therefore, in a state of balance that can be lost with ligamentous injury or fracture. Biomechanical studies have shown that wrist ligament injury propagates in predictable patterns, potentially creating perilunate or lunate dislocations. Because of the unique material properties of the intrinsic wrist ligaments, anatomic restoration of the acutely disrupted carpal ligament is the usual goal of surgery.

References

1. Mikic ZD: Arthrography of the wrist joint: An experimental study. *J Bone Joint Surg Am* 1984;66:371-378.
2. An KN, Berger RA, Cooney WP (eds): *Biomechanics of the Wrist Joint.* New York, NY, Springer-Verlag, 1991.
3. Smith DK, Cooney WP III, An KN, Linscheid RL, Chao EY: The effects of simulated unstable scaphoid fractures on carpal motion. *J Hand Surg Am* 1989;14:283-291.
4. Berger RA, Crowninshield RD, Flatt AE: The three-dimensional rotational behaviors of the carpal bones. *Clin Orthop* 1982;167:303-310.
5. Garcia-Elias M, Cooney WP, An KN, Linscheid RL, Chao EY: Wrist kinematics after limited intercarpal arthrodesis. *J Hand Surg Am* 1989;14:791-799.
6. Horii E, Garcia-Elias M, An KN, et al: A kinematic study of luno-triquetral dissociations. *J Hand Surg Am* 1991;16:355-362.
7. Ruby LK, An KN, Linscheid RL, Cooney WP III, Chao EY: The effect of scapholunate ligament section on scapholunate motion. *J Hand Surg Am* 1987;12:767-771.
8. Destot EAJ (ed): *Injuries of the Wrist: A Radiologic Study.* New York, NY, Paul B Hoeber, 1926.
9. Navarro A: Luxaciones del carpo. *An Fac Med Montevideo* 1921;6:113-141.
10. Gilford WW, Bolton RH, Lambrinudi C: The mechanism of the wrist joint: With special reference to fractures of the scaphoid. *Guy's Hosp Rep* 1943;92:52-59.
11. Fisk GR: Carpal instability and the fractured scaphoid. *Ann R Coll Surg Engl* 1970;46:63-76.
12. Linscheid RL, Dobyns JH, Beabout JW, Bryan RS: Traumatic instability of the wrist: Diagnosis, classification, and pathomechanics. *J Bone Joint Surg Am* 1972;54:1612-1632.
13. Linscheid RL, Dobyns JH, Beckenbaugh RD, Cooney WP III, Wood MB: Instability patterns of the wrist. *J Hand Surg Am* 1983;8:682-686.
14. Linscheid RL, Dobyns JH: The unified concept of carpal injuries. *Ann Chir Main* 1984;3:35-42.
15. Mayfield JK, Johnson RP, Kilcoyne RF: The ligaments of the human wrist and their functional significance. *Anat Rec* 1976;186:417-428.
16. Mayfield JK, Johnson RP, Kilcoyne RK: Carpal dislocations: Pathomechanics and progressive perilunar instability. *J Hand Surg Am* 1980;5:226-241.
17. Mayfield JK: Mechanism of carpal injuries. *Clin Orthop* 1980;149:45-54.
18. Taleisnik J: Triquetrohamate and triquetrolunate instabilities (medial carpal instability). *Ann Chir Main* 1984;3:331-343.
19. Taleisnik J, Watson HK: Midcarpal instability caused by malunited fractures of the distal radius. *J Hand Surg Am* 1984;9:350-357.
20. Taleisnik J: Carpal instability. *J Bone Joint Surg Am* 1988;70:1262-1268.
21. Lichtman DM, Bruckner JD, Culp RW, Alexander CE: Palmar midcarpal instability: Results of surgical reconstruction. *J Hand Surg Am* 1993;18:307-315.
22. Lichtman DM, Noble WH III, Alexander CE: Dynamic triquetrolunate instability: Case report. *J Hand Surg Am* 1984;9:185-188.
23. Lichtman DM, Schneider JR, Swafford AR, Mack GR: Ulnar midcarpal instability: Clinical and laboratory analysis. *J Hand Surg Am* 1981;6:515-523.
24. Watson H, Ottoni L, Pitts EC, Handal AG: Rotary subluxation of the scaphoid: A spectrum of instability. *J Hand Surg Br* 1993;18:62-64.
25. Watson HK, Belniak R, Garcia-Elias M: Treatment of scapholunate dissociation: Preferred treatment: STT fusion vs other methods. *Orthopedics* 1991;14:365-370.
26. Watson HK, Ryu J, Akelman E: Limited triscaphoid intercarpal arthrodesis for rotatory subluxation of the scaphoid. *J Bone Joint Surg Am* 1986;68:345-349.
27. Andrews JG, Youm Y: A biomechanical investigation of wrist kinematics. *J Biomech* 1979;12:83-93.
28. Youm Y, Yoon YS: Analytical development in investigation of wrist kinematics. *J Biomech* 1979;12:613-621.
29. McMurtry RY, Youm Y, Flatt AE, Gillespie TE: Kinematics of the wrist: II. Clinical applications. *J Bone Joint Surg Am* 1978;60:955-961.

30. Youm Y, McMurtry RY, Flatt AE, Gillespie TE: Kinematics of the wrist: I. An experimental study of radial-ulnar deviation and flexion-extension. *J Bone Joint Surg Am* 1978;60:423-431.

31. de Lange A, Kauer JM, Huiskes R: Kinematic behavior of the human wrist joint: A roentgen-stereophotogrammetric analysis. *J Orthop Res* 1985;3:56-64.

32. Savelberg HH, Kooloos JG, De Lange A, Huiskes R, Kauer JM: Human carpal ligament recruitment and three-dimensional carpal motion. *J Orthop Res* 1991;9:693-704.

33. Ritt MJ, Berger RA, Kauer JM: The gross and histologic anatomy of the ligaments of the capitohamate joint. *J Hand Surg Am* 1996;21:1022-1028.

34. Ritt MJ, Berger RA, Bishop AT, An KN: The capitohamate ligaments: A comparison of biomechanical properties. *J Hand Surg Br* 1996;21:451-454.

35. Kauer JM: The mechanism of the carpal joint. *Clin Orthop* 1986:202:16-26.

36. Berger RA: The anatomy and basic biomechanics of the wrist joint. *J Hand Ther* 1996;9:84-93.

37. Berger RA, Imeada T, Berglund L, An KN: Constraint and material properties of the subregions of the scapholunate interosseous ligament. *J Hand Surg Am* 1999;24:953-962.

38. Trumble TE, Bour CJ, Smith RJ, Glisson RR: Kinematics of the ulnar carpus related to the volar intercalated segment instability pattern. *J Hand Surg Am* 1990;15:384-392.

39. Viegas SF, Patterson RM, Peterson PD, et al: Ulnar-sided perilunate instability: An anatomic and biomechanic study. *J Hand Surg Am* 1990;15:268-278.

40. Ruby LK, Cooney WP III, An KN, Linscheid RL, Chao EY: Relative motion of selected carpal bones: A kinematic analysis of the normal wrist. *J Hand Surg Am* 1988;13:1-10.

41. Sennwald GR, Zdravkovic V, Jacob HA, Kern HP: Kinematic analysis of relative motion within the proximal carpal row. *J Hand Surg Br* 1993;18:609-612.

42. Amadio PC: Carpal kinematics and instability: A clinical and anatomic primer. *Clin Anat* 1991;4:1-12.

43. Sarrafian SK, Melamed JL, Goshgarian GM: Study of wrist motion in flexion and extension. *Clin Orthop* 1977;126:153-159.

44. Kauer JM: The interdependence of carpal articulation chains. *Acta Anat* 1974;88:481-501.

45. Brahin B, Allieu Y: Compensatory carpal malalignments. *Ann Chir Main* 1984;3:357-363.

46. Allieu Y, Brahin B, Asencio G: Carpal instabilities: Radiological and clinico-pathological classification. *Ann Radiol* 1982;25:275-287.

47. Mouchet A, Belot J: Poignet a ressaut (subluxation mediocarpienne en avant). *Bull Mem Soc Nat Chir* 1934;60:1243-1244.

48. Reagan DS, Linscheid RL, Dobyns JH: Lunotriquetral sprains. *J Hand Surg Am* 1984;9:502-514.

49. Wright TW, Dobyns JH, Linscheid RL, Macksoud W, Siegert J: Carpal instability non-dissociative. *J Hand Surg Br* 1994;19:763-773.

50. Johnson RP, Carrera GF: Chronic capitolunate instability. *J Bone Joint Surg Am* 1986;68:1164-1176.

51. Garcia-Elias M, Dobyns JH, Cooney WP III, Linscheid RL: Traumatic axial dislocations of the carpus. *J Hand Surg Am* 1989;14:446-457.

52. Garcia-Elias M, An KN, Cooney WP, Linscheid RL, Chao EY: Transverse stability of the carpus: An analytical study. *J Orthop Res* 1989;7:738-743.

53. Garcia-Elias M, An KN, Cooney WP III, Linscheid RL, Chao EY: Stability of the transverse carpal arch: An experimental study. *J Hand Surg Am* 1989;14:277-282.

54. Linscheid RL, Dobyns JH: Carpal instability. *Curr Orthop* 1989;3:106-114.

55. Taleisnik J: Post-traumatic carpal instability. *Clin Orthop* 1980;149:73-82.

56. Green DP, O'Brien ET: Classification and management of carpal dislocations. *Clin Orthop* 1980;149:55-72.

57. Louis DS, Hankin FM, Greene TL: Letter. Chronic capitolunate instability. *J Bone Joint Surg Am* 1987;69:950-951.

58. Cooney WP III, Linscheid RL, Dobyns JH: Fractures and dislocations of the wrist, in Rockwood CA Jr, Green DP, Bucholz RW, Heckman JD (eds): *Rockwood and Green's Fractures in Adults,* ed 4. Philadelphia, PA, Lippincott-Raven, 1996, pp 745-867.

59. Frank C, Woo S, Andriacchi T, et al: Normal ligament: Structure, function, and composition, in Woo SLY, Buckwalter JA (eds): *Injury and Repair of the Musculoskeletal Soft Tissues.* Park Ridge, IL, American Academy of Orthopaedic Surgeons, 1988, pp 45-101.

60. Berger RA: General anatomy, in Cooney WP, Linscheid RL, Dobyns JH (eds): *The Wrist: Diagnosis and Operative Treatment.* St Louis, MO, Mosby-Year Book, 1998, pp 32-60.

61. Mayfield JK, Williams WJ, Erdman AG, et al: Biomechanical properties of human carpal ligaments. *Orthop Trans* 1979;3:143-144.

62. Nowak MD: Material properties of ligaments, in An K-N, Berger RA, Cooney WP III (eds): *Biomechanics of the Wrist Joint.* New York, NY, Springer-Verlag, 1991, pp 139-156.

63. Berger RA, Kauer JM, Landsmeer JM: Radioscapholunate ligament: A gross anatomic and histologic study of fetal and adult wrists. *J Hand Surg Am* 1991;16:350-355.

64. Logan SE, Nowak MD: Intrinsic and extrinsic wrist ligaments: Biomechanical and functional differences. *Biomed Sci Instrum* 1987;23:9-13.

65. Berger RA: The gross and histologic anatomy of the scapholunate interosseous ligament. *J Hand Surg Am* 1996;21:170-178.

66. Berger R, Imeada T, Berglund L, et al: The anatomic, constraint and material properties of the scapholunate interosseous ligament: A preliminary, in Schuind F, An KN, Cooney WP, et al (eds): *Advances in the Biomechanics of the Hand and Wrist.* New York, NY, Plenum Press, 1994, pp 9-17.

67. Mayfield JK: Wrist ligamentous anatomy and pathogenesis of carpal instability. *Orthop Clin North Am* 1984;15: 209-216.

68. Mayfield JK: Patterns of injury to carpal ligaments: A spectrum. *Clin Orthop* 1984;187:36-42.

69. Johnson RP: The acutely injured wrist and its residuals. *Clin Orthop* 1980;149:33-44.

70. Bishop AT, Reagan, DS: Lunotriquetral sprains, in Cooney WP, Linscheid RL, Dobyns JH (eds): *The Wrist: Diagnosis and Operative Treatment.* St Louis, MO, Mosby-Year Book, 1998, pp 527-549.

71. Smith DK, Murray PM: Avulsion fractures of the volar aspect of triquetral bone of the wrist: A subtle sign of carpal ligament injury. *AJR Am J Roentgenol* 1996;166:609-614.

72. Palmer C, Murray PM, et al: The mechanism of ulnar-sided perilunar instability of the wrist. *Fourteenth Annual Meeting of the Southern Orthopaedic Association.* Pebble Beach, CA, 1998.

73. Cooney WP, Bussey R, Dobyns JH, Linscheid RL: Difficult wrist fractures: Perilunate fracture-dislocations of the wrist. *Clin Orthop* 1987;214:136-147.

74. Norbeck DE Jr, Larson B, Blair SJ, Demos TC: Traumatic longitudinal disruption of the carpus. *J Hand Surg Am* 1987;12:509-514.

75. Green DP, O'Brien ET: Open reduction of carpal dislocations: Indications and operative techniques. *J Hand Surg Am* 1978;3:250-265.

76. Primiano GA, Reef TC: Disruption of the proximal carpal arch of the hand. *J Bone Joint Surg Am* 1974;56:328-332.

77. Garcia-Elias M, Abanco J, Salvador E, Sanchez R: Crush injury of the carpus. *J Bone Joint Surg Br* 1985;67:286-289.

78. Shin AY, Glowacki KA, Bishop AT: Dynamic axial carpal instability: A case report. *J Hand Surg Am* 1999;24:781-785.

79. Chow SP: Moulding press injury of the hand. *Ann Acad Med Singapore* 1979;8:493-496.

80. Chow SP, So YC, Pun WK, Luk KD, Leong JC: Thenar crush injuries. *J Bone Joint Surg Br* 1988;70:135-139.

81. Matev I: Wringer injuries of the hand. *J Bone Joint Surg Br* 1967;49:722-730.

82. Lavernia CJ, Cohen MS, Taleisnik J: Treatment of scapholunate dissociation by ligamentous repair and capsulodesis. *J Hand Surg Am* 1992;17:354-359.

83. Sotereanos DG, Mitsionis GJ, Giannakopoulos PN, Tomaino MM, Herndon JH: Perilunate dislocation and fracture dislocation: A critical analysis of the volar-dorsal approach. *J Hand Surg Am* 1997;22:49-56.

84. Herzberg G, Comtet JJ, Linscheid RL, Amadio PC, Cooney WP, Stadler J: Perilunate dislocations and fracture-dislocations: A multicenter study. *J Hand Surg Am* 1993;18:768-779.

CHAPTER 3

DIAGNOSIS OF ACUTE CARPAL LIGAMENT INJURIES

PHILIP E. BLAZAR, MD
JEFFREY N. LAWTON, MD

Injuries to the ligaments of the wrist represent a broad spectrum of pathology. Accurate diagnosis and treatment of these injuries is complicated by the complex anatomy due to the large number of intrinsic and extrinsic ligaments in the wrist. In addition, without using invasive techniques, the ability to directly stress or visualize individual ligaments is limited. Therefore, injuries to these structures may be suspected but can rarely be proven conclusively with routine examination and radiographs. Ligament injuries are often implied by gross radiographic alterations; but wrist instability patterns frequently present only after some time has elapsed. This chapter focuses on diagnosis of the more common acute carpal ligament injuries, including the use of imaging modalities.

CLASSIFICATION

Wrist ligament injuries are classified by radiographic pattern, behavior, and chronicity. The patterns of instability are changes produced within the carpus by ligamentous or bony disruptions. The classification of Linscheid and associates[1] is based primarily on the position of the lunate and the capitolunate angle as seen on a lateral radiograph. An instability pattern is termed a dorsal intercalated segment instability (DISI) if the lunate is abnormally extended (>15° for the capitolunate angle and >60° for the scapholunate angle) and palmarly translated with the capitate subluxated dorsal to the long axis of the radius. A volar intercalated segment instability (VISI) pattern is an abnormally flexed (>30° for the capitolunate angle or <30° for the scapholunate angle) and dorsally translated lunate with the capitate subluxated palmar to the long axis of the radius (Fig. 1).

Patterns of instability can be further described based on the normal patterns of motion. Both the proximal and distal carpal rows have particular patterns of motion within the rows (ie, relationship of the scaphoid relative to the lunate). This normal motion has been termed "associative." A disruption of the normal kinematics within a row is a dissociative instability (Fig. 2); a disruption between rows, while the alignment within each row remains normal, is a nondissociative instability. Dissociative carpal instabilities may result from a disruption of any of the bony or ligamentous components of the wrist.

Taleisnik[2] introduced the concept of static and dynamic instability. A static instability is diagnosed when standard wrist radiographs reveal evidence of abnormal carpal alignment. With a dynamic instability, in contrast, radiographs reveal abnormal carpal alignment only when a stress is applied (eg, a clenched-fist view) or when the wrist is in a nonstandard position. Dynamic and static instability can be thought of as different stages in a clinical spectrum of partial to complete ligament injury. Frequently, but not exclusively, nondissociative instabilities are dynamic at presentation, and dissociative instabilities are static.

Instability patterns also may be adaptive, secondary to changes outside the carpus such as a VISI deformity with a distal radius malunion. They also may be complex combinations of dissociative, nondissociative, and axial instabilities.

As noted in chapter 2, Mayfield and associates[3] have described four stages of ligament disruption in progressive perilunate instability: stage I, scapholunate; stage II, capitolunate; stage III, triquetrolunate; and stage IV, radiolunate. Murray and associates (Minneapolis, MN, unpublished data, 1998) have described a similar sequence of injuries to the

FIGURE 1

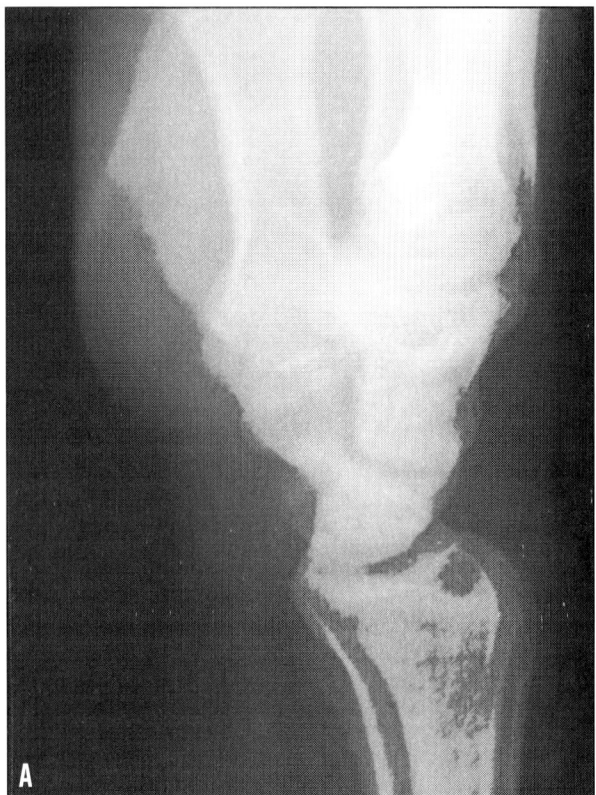 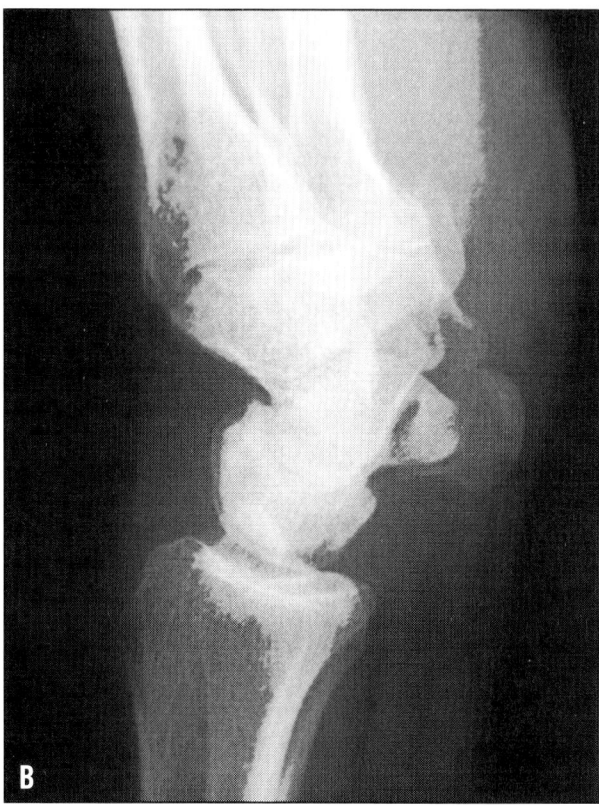

A, Lateral radiograph of a right wrist showing a dorsal intercalated segment instability (DISI) pattern in a patient with a scapholunate dissociation. Note that the lunate is tilted dorsally and the long axis of the capitate is displaced dorsal to the long axis of the radius. **B,** Lateral radiograph of a left wrist showing a volar intercalated segment instability (VISI) pattern in a patient with a midcarpal instability. Note that the lunate is tilted palmarly and the long axis of the capitate is displaced palmar to the long axis of the radius.

ulnar side of the carpus, although these are much less common. Many of these injuries occur in association with fractures of one or more carpal bones. This has led to the concept of lesser arc and greater arc injuries (Fig. 3).

PATIENT EVALUATION

The etiologies of wrist ligament injuries range from high-energy polytrauma to low-energy mechanisms that cause mild, protracted symptoms. Wrist ligament injuries can range from subtle instability patterns as the result of attrition to acute and chronic injuries. Evaluation for wrist ligament injuries and resultant instability is mandatory in all patients with wrist symptoms, whether or not a recent traumatic event is identified. Even gross carpal malalignment (eg, perilunate dislocations) may be overlooked or misdiagnosed at the time of initial injury and radiographic

examination. The most devastating of these injuries, lunate or perilunate dislocations, comprise only 10% of all carpal injuries and usually occur as a result of high-energy injuries.[4] Of these, transscaphoid perilunate fracture-dislocations are the most common, representing 61% of all perilunate dislocations in one study (Fig. 4).

The evaluation begins with a thorough, directed history including age, hand dominance, the nature of injury, occupational and recreational history, onset of symptoms, loss of motion, prior hand or wrist conditions, and past medical history. All of these components of a patient's history can influence treatment decisions.

In the acute high-energy injury, physical examination may reveal gross deformity, swelling, ecchymosis, or lacerations. Carpal injury may be overlooked or considered a low priority in this setting. Range-of-motion testing, palpation for specific sites of tenderness, and a careful

FIGURE 2

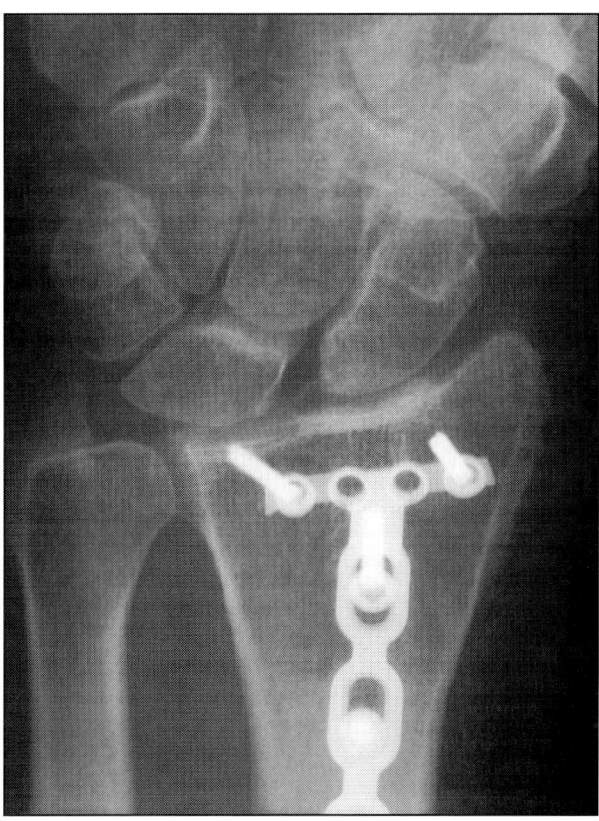

A scapholunate ligament tear (dissociative instability) seen in association with a distal radius fracture (healed).

FIGURE 3

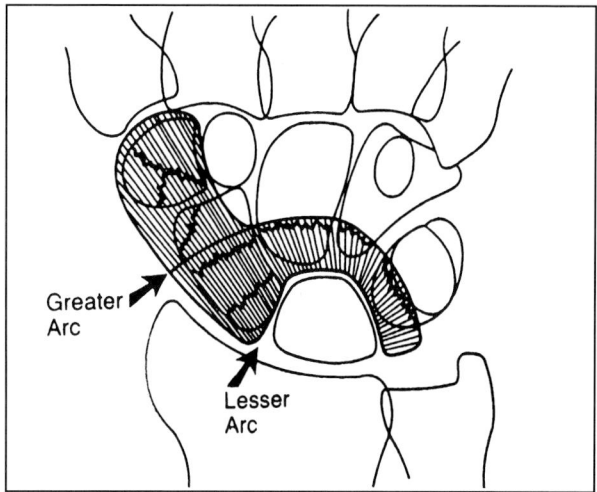

Diagram depicting greater and lesser arc injuries. Greater arc injuries include disruption of bony elements, whereas lesser arc injuries affect ligamentous structures.

neurologic/vascular examination, especially with sensory testing, are mandatory. In one study,[5] perilunate dislocations were associated with up to 25% of the cases of acute carpal tunnel syndrome.

Patients with injuries caused by subacute or chronic processes may present with pain, popping, catching, or symptoms of secondary degenerative changes. In these patients, a more detailed examination of the carpus is performed. Active and passive range of motion are assessed and recorded. Identifying specific areas of tenderness is frequently the most helpful portion of the examination in localizing the diagnosis. The bony components of the carpus are all palpable, so direct palpation over the scapholunate, lunotriquetral, triangular fibrocartilage complex, and midcarpal joints may greatly narrow the differential diagnosis.

Specific maneuvers to check for ligamentous disruption of the wrist may also help determine the extent of the injury. A systematic approach, beginning on the radial

aspect of the wrist, can help with the evaluation. This approach would begin with Watson's scaphoid shift test, followed by the midcarpal shuck test and the lunotriquetral ballottement test. The scaphoid shift test is performed by placing pressure on the scaphoid tubercle with the examiner's index finger as the wrist is brought from radial to ulnar deviation. If the scaphoid lunate interosseous ligament has been disrupted, a clunking occurs as the proximal pole of the scaphoid slams into the dorsal rim of the radius. The midcarpal shuck test is performed by pressing on the dorsal surface of the capitate as the wrist is moved from radial to ulnar deviation. There is normally a gentle snap as the lunate "catches up" and rotates dorsally. When midcarpal instability is present, there is a pronounced clunk as the lunate reduces from its palmar flexed position. The scaphoid shift (Fig. 5) and midcarpal shuck maneuvers both reproduce an abnormal wrist subluxation suggestive of ligament disruption.[6,7] Lunotriquetral ballottement (Fig. 6) and shearing maneuvers stress this articulation, thus reproducing symptoms in patients with lunotriquetral instability or arthritis.[7,8] In the subacute, or low-energy, injury, it is important to assess the contralateral wrist for these same signs, as ligamentous laxity varies widely between individuals. A symmetric positive maneuver with a unilateral injury is a much less specific finding.

Recently, a number of authors have highlighted the association of wrist ligament injuries with distal radius

FIGURE 4

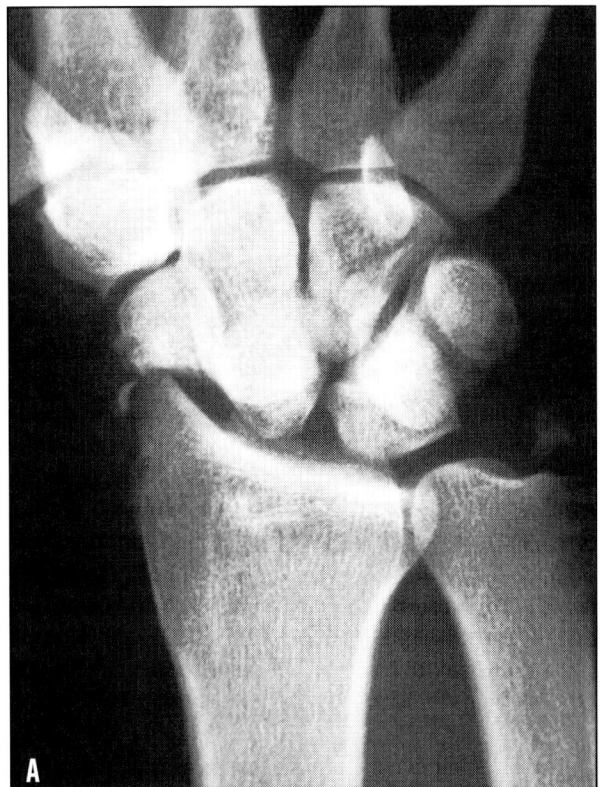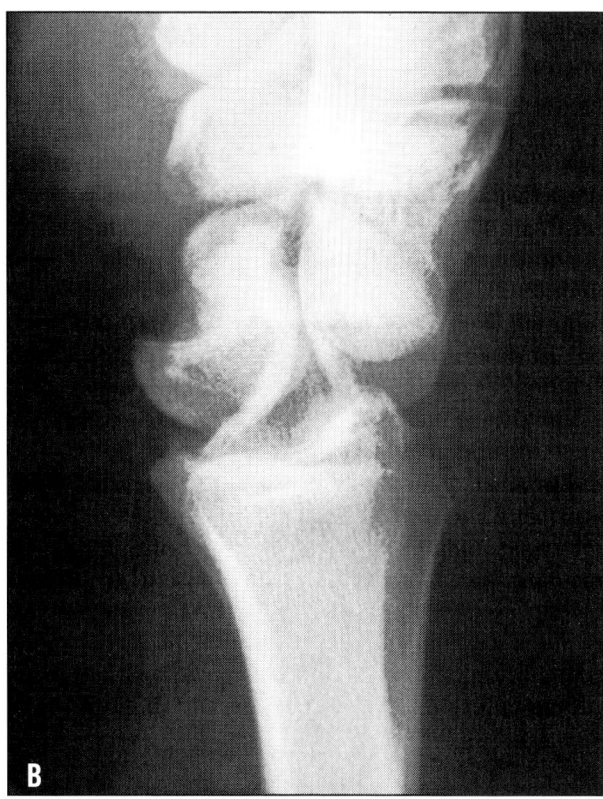

A transscaphoid perilunate variant prior to reduction. **A,** PA radiograph. **B,** Lateral radiograph.

fractures[9] (Fig. 2). One study based on arthroscopic evaluation found an incidence of 78%. However, the clinical significance of these injuries remains unclear.[7]

IMAGING

Imaging modalities used in the diagnosis of suspected acute carpal ligament injuries include radiography, CT, arthrography, fluoroscopy, scintigraphy, and MRI. At the very minimum, plain radiographs must be obtained. These are most helpful when setting fractures or diagnosing ligament disruption with associated fractures. The use of other modalities must be based on the particular clinical scenario. Many of these tests produce a high frequency of abnormal findings in asymptomatic wrists and therefore should be avoided unless they are clearly indicated to correlate with specific symptoms. Unnecessary tests may obfuscate the diagnosis with "abnormal" findings that are not germane to the patient's condition.

Plain Radiographs and Fluoroscopy

Radiographic examination of the wrist is mandatory in all suspected wrist ligament injuries and instabilities. PA, lateral, and oblique radiographs constitute a standard wrist trauma series. Gilula[10] has described normal carpal alignment on the PA view as consisting of three parallel carpal arcs (Fig. 7). Disruption of one of these arcs suggests either a fracture or subluxation from a ligamentous injury. Increased distance between the scaphoid and lunate may indicate scapholunate interosseous ligament disruption. With lunotriquetral ligament tears, proximal translation of the triquetrum seen on the PA view is more common, but the lunotriquetral distance does not typically increase. In patients with acute, gross malalignment of the carpus, a PA radiograph with 5 to 10 lb of traction frequently aids in assessment of intracarpal ligament disruptions or fractures. Lateral radiographs should be carefully evaluated to make sure that the capitate reduces in the lunate and the lunate is reduced in the fossa of the

FIGURE 5

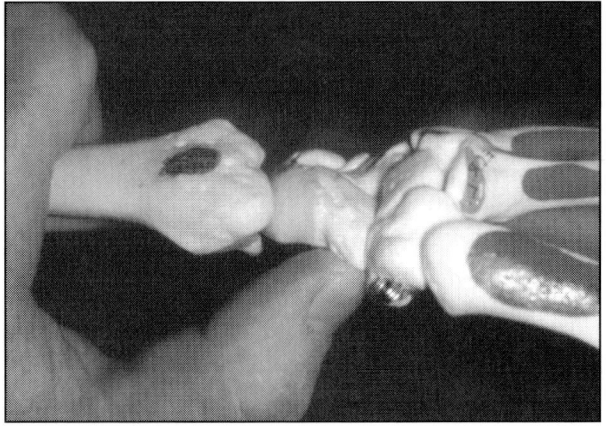

The scaphoid shift test is performed with the examiner's thumb on the scaphoid tubercle. The wrist is brought from ulnar to radial deviation while the examiner applies dorsally directed pressure to the scaphoid. The pathologic finding is a "clunk" with subluxation of the scaphoid dorsally out of the scaphoid fossa. (Reproduced from Light TR (ed): *Hand Surgery Update 2*. Rosemont, IL, American Academy of Orthopaedic Surgeons, 1999, p 99.)

FIGURE 6

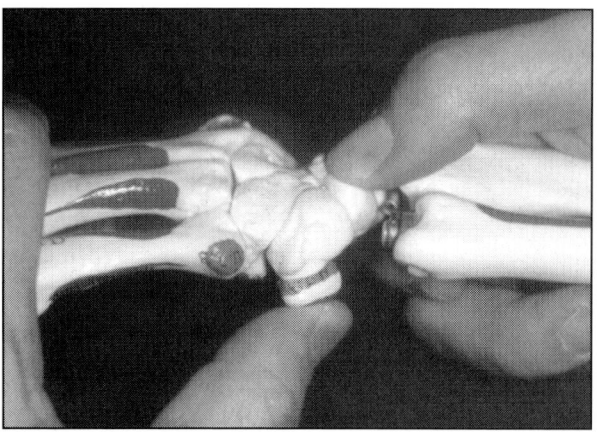

Lunotriquetral ballottement is performed by fixing the lunate with the thumb (and index finger) of one hand and displacing the triquetrum palmarly and dorsally with the thumb of the other hand. A positive result is pain elicited with the maneuver. (Reproduced from Light TR (ed): *Hand Surgery Update 2*. Rosemont, IL, American Academy of Orthopaedic Surgeons, 1999, p 100.)

radius. A significant number of perilunate dislocations are missed because the radiographs are not carefully reviewed and correlated with clinical findings.

Although the lateral radiograph may be more difficult to interpret than a PA view because many of the carpal bones overlap on this view, many patterns of instability can be identified. Radiolunate, capitolunate, scapholunate, and lunotriquetral angles may all be calculated from the lateral radiograph and compared to published norms (Fig. 8). DISI is defined as a scapholunate angle > 60° (mean, 45°; range, 38° to 60°) with a capitolunate angle > 30° (mean, 0°; range, 30° dorsal to 30° palmar). VISI is defined as a scapholunate angle < 30°. In many acute carpal ligament disruptions, the initial plain radiographs are normal, with instability patterns recognized only as a late finding.

Specific instability views may be indicated to accentuate more subtle instabilities; for example, a PA clenched-fist view can demonstrate dynamic scapholunate widening. Some authors recommend radiographs with traction to accentuate these instabilities. At least 20 instability views have been described. When a full wrist instability series is indicated, it is frequently helpful to use fluoroscopy while reproducing a subluxation maneuver. Fluoroscopy or cineradiographic examination with provocative motion or maneuvers can demonstrate dynamic instability.

Computed Tomography

Trispiral CT has been used in a limited manner for acute carpal injuries. CT of both wrists in pronation, neutral, and supination has become the study of choice to evaluate the distal radioulnar joint for subluxation or dislocation. CT provides more detailed evaluation of bony anatomy than do radiographs and may be indicated for subtle intra-articular fractures, to assess the degree of displacement, or to check for union of a fracture. CT has been used increasingly in recent years to assess scaphoid fractures for comminution, displacement, and fracture pattern.

Bone Scintigraphy

Technetium Tc 99m bone scans identify varying levels of bone remodeling. With acute wrist injury, these studies may be helpful to identify radiographically occult fractures, most commonly those of the scaphoid. A focal area of increased uptake may suggest a fracture or a ligament injury. As with other musculoskeletal sites, bone scans of the carpus are sensitive but not specific.

Arthrography

Arthrography has historically been the gold standard diagnostic test for evaluating ligament disruption of the carpus. Contrast medium is injected into the radiocarpal,

FIGURE 7

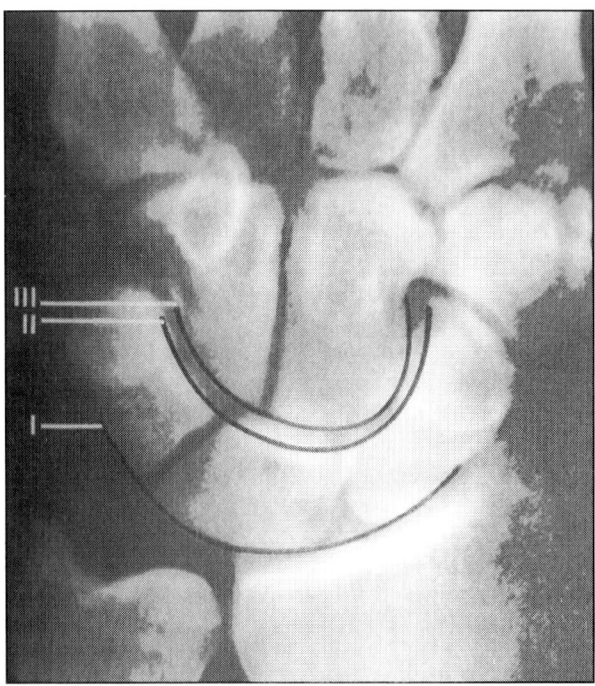

Carpal arcs described by Gilula.[10]

FIGURE 8

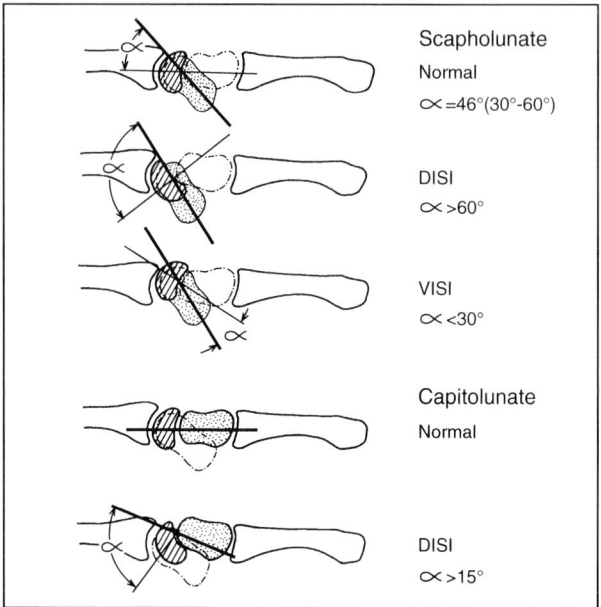

Scapholunate and capitolunate angles in the normal hand and in the presence of instability. (Reproduced with permission from Trumble TE: Fractures and dislocations of the carpus, in Trumble TE: *Principles of Hand Surgery and Therapy.* Philadelphia, PA, WB Saunders, 2000, p 91.)

midcarpal, and radioulnar compartments, with dye flow between any two indicating a tear. The three-compartment injection is less time-consuming than the triple injection technique, which requires a time interval for clearance between injections. In general, arthrography in the acute setting is utilized to evaluate the triangular fibrocartilage complex and the lunotriquetral and scapholunate interosseous ligaments. Arthrography lacks specificity, is an invasive procedure, and provides no information on the chronicity or etiology of the communications. Because the results of arthrography must therefore be carefully correlated with clinical findings, its most common use tends to be for evaluation of subacute or chronic wrist symptoms. Metz and associates[11] found a low correlation between symptoms and the location of wrist ligament injuries as revealed by arthrography.[10] Arthrography can be combined with videotaped motion sequences, which provide additional information about carpal kinematic alterations. A high incidence of bilateral defects is found in patients with unilateral symptoms.[12,13] Many authors strongly suggest bilateral arthrography to check for asymmetry of communicating defects as a means of increasing specificity.

Magnetic Resonance Imaging

MRI has gained in popularity for evaluation of the carpus as examiners have become more experienced. It is a noninvasive modality with the potential to provide diagnostic evaluation of intrinsic and extrinsic carpal ligaments as well as the carpal bones. MRI has the advantage of providing diagnostic information for a variety of other soft-tissue and bony pathologies about the wrist such as ganglia, bone or soft-tissue tumors, and osteonecrosis. However, the small size of many of the intrinsic wrist ligaments can make them difficult to routinely image. The information obtained, however, is very dependent on the equipment used and the skill of the radiologist. Potter and associates[14] have shown a specificity of 90% and a sensitivity of 100% for evaluation of triangular fibrocartilage complex tears, although not all authors have found similar results. Some investigators are exploring the diagnostic utility of MR arthrography with injection of gadolinium as a contrast medium to enhance accuracy rates.

Arthroscopy

Because of the limited sensitivity and specificity of less invasive modalities, diagnostic arthroscopy plays a sub-

TABLE 1

Arthroscopic Classification of Tears of the Intracarpal Ligaments

Grade	Description
I	Attenuation or hemorrhage of the interosseous ligament as seen from the radiocarpal space. No incongruency of carpal alignment in the midcarpal space.
II	Attenuation or hemorrhage of the interosseous ligament as seen from the radiocarpal space. Incongruency or step-off of carpal space. There may be a slight gap (less than the width of a probe) between carpal bones.
III	Incongruency or step-off of carpal alignment as seen from both radiocarpal and midcarpal space. Probe may be passed through gap between carpal bones.
IV	Incongruency or step-off of carpal alignment as seen from both radiocarpal and midcarpal space. There is gross instability with manipulation. A 2.7-mm arthroscope may be passed through the gap between carpal bones.

(Reproduced with permission from Geissler WB, Freeland AE, Savioe FH, McIntyre LW, Whipple TL: Intracarpal soft-tissue lesions associated with an intra-articular fracture of the distal end of the radius. *J Bone Joint Surg Am* 1996;78:357-365.)

SUMMARY

The diagnosis of acute carpal ligament injuries continues to evolve. In cases of gross malalignment, such as a perilunate dislocation, the ligamentous disruptions are evaluated at the time of surgical repair. Thus, imaging beyond plain radiographs, either with or without traction, is not required. With a more subtle disruption of the carpus, a variety of studies may be indicated. The primary modality for establishing the diagnosis of carpal ligament tears, however, remains the physical examination. Wrist arthroscopy remains the gold standard for evaluating carpal ligaments and continues to play a prominent role as a diagnostic modality in complex situations.

REFERENCES

1. Linscheid RL, Dobyns JH, Beabout JW, Bryan RS: Traumatic instability of the wrist: Diagnosis, classification, and pathomechanics. *J Bone Joint Surg Am* 1972;54:1612-1632.
2. Taleisnik J: Post-traumatic carpal instability. *Clin Orthop* 1980;149:73-82.
3. Mayfield JK, Johnson RP, Kilcoyne RK: Carpal dislocations: Pathomechanics and progressive perilunar instability. *J Hand Surg Am* 1980;5:226-241.
4. Minami A, Kaneda K: Repair and/or reconstruction of scapholunate interosseous ligament in lunate and perilunate dislocations. *J Hand Surg Am* 1993;18:1099-1106.
5. Herzberg G, Comtet JJ, Linscheid RL, Amadio PC, Cooney WP, Stadler J: Perilunate dislocations and fracture-dislocations: A multicenter study. *J Hand Surg Am* 1993;18:768-779.
6. Lichtman DM, Schneider JR, Swafford AR, Mack GR: Ulnar midcarpal instability: Clinical and laboratory analysis. *J Hand Surg Am* 1981;6:515-523.
7. Watson HK, Weinzweig J: Physical examination of the wrist. *Hand Clin* 1997;13:17-34.
8. Reagan DS, Linscheid RL, Dobyns JH: Lunotriquetral sprains. *J Hand Surg Am* 1984;9:502-514.
9. Lindau T, Arner M, Hagberg L: Intraarticular lesions in distal fractures of the radius in young adults: A descriptive arthroscopic study in 50 patients. *J Hand Surg Br* 1997;22:638-643.
10. Gilula LA: Imaging and evaluation, in *Hand Surgery Update 2*. Rosemont, IL, American Academy of Orthopaedic Surgeons, 1994, pp 63-76.
11. Metz VM, Mann FA, Gilula LA: Lack of correlation between site of wrist pain and location of noncommunicating defects shown by three-compartment wrist arthrography. *AJR Am J Roentgenol* 1993;160:1239-1243.

stantial role in the evaluation of the carpal ligaments, especially in isolated ligament tears. Wrist arthroscopy also has the potential to provide therapeutic modalities for carpal ligament injuries. Although many authors still prefer open repairs of many complete ligament disruptions,[15] arthroscopy is currently considered the gold standard for evaluation of ligament disruptions. The technique affords the surgeon the opportunity to visualize, probe, and stress intrinsic and extrinsic carpal ligaments. Arthroscopic grading of ligament disruptions may help the surgeon select a treatment modality (Table 1). Arthroscopy may be indicated to rule out an acute ligamentous disruption such as an acute scapholunate tear or to evaluate the carpus more extensively when there are subtle signs of carpal instability. Arthroscopy is a very sensitive diagnostic test, and frequently clinically silent lesions may be detected. However, as a therapeutic modality, arthroscopy currently has limited indications in carpal fractures and dislocations, and it is an invasive technique requiring anesthesia.

12. Kirschenbaum D, Sieler S, Solonick D, Loeb DM, Cody RP: Arthrography of the wrist: Assessment of the integrity of the ligaments in young asymptomatic adults. *J Bone Joint Surg Am* 1995;77:1207-1209.

13. Yin YM, Evanoff B, Gilula LA, Pilgram TK: Evaluation of selective wrist arthrography of contralateral asymptomatic wrists for symmetric ligamentous defects. *AJR Am J Roentgenol* 1996;166:1067-1073.

14. Potter HG, Asnis-Ernberg L, Weiland AJ, Hotchkiss RN, Peterson MG, McCormack RR Jr: The utility of high-resolution magnetic resonance imaging in the evaluation of the triangular fibrocartilage complex of the wrist. *J Bone Joint Surg Am* 1997;79:1675-1684.

15. Stanley JK, Trail IA: Carpal instability. *J Bone Joint Surg Br* 1994;76:691-700.

CHAPTER 4

LUNATE AND PERILUNATE DISLOCATIONS

DUC P. VO, MD

L. RANDALL MOHLER, MD

THOMAS E. TRUMBLE, MD

C arpal dislocations are rare, complex injuries. Nearly every imaginable combination of radiocarpal and intercarpal dislocation has been described, and few fit neatly into a particular pattern or classification scheme. The injury may be subtle both clinically and radiographically, and diagnosis is frequently delayed. Prompt recognition, accurate reduction, and stable temporary internal fixation all contribute to improved outcomes.

Because the lunate is strongly bound to the radius and ulna by the palmar capsular ligaments, in severe injuries the lunate often remains reduced to the distal radius while the remainder of the carpus is dislocated. These injuries are commonly referred to as perilunate dislocations.

Lunate dislocations occur when the lunate rotates palmarly on these strong capsular ligaments and the remainder of the carpus and hand remains relatively aligned with the distal radius and ulna. Both injuries lie within the spectrum of fracture-dislocations of the carpus (Fig. 1). Perilunate dislocations and lunate dislocations may represent stages of a common spectrum of injury and are typically considered together. For the purpose of this discussion, both patterns generally will be considered as perilunate injuries. Perilunate injuries are frequently divided into dislocations and fracture-dislocations. Pure dislocations are relatively less common; careful intraoperative inspection of these injuries frequently reveals chondral or osteochondral injuries not apparent on radiographs. This chapter focuses on the evaluation and management of lunate and perilunate dislocations.

HISTORICAL PERSPECTIVE

Perilunate dislocations comprise a broad continuum of injuries ranging from minor ligament strains to complete dislocation of the lunate. The earliest written subject matter on these particular injuries, associated with carpal instabilities in general, was Destot's 1926 work.[1] In the 1920s, as reports of lunate dislocations began to appear, methods for closed reduction were proposed. Also in the 1920s, Gunn's law was formulated. This law, which states that a deformity should be recreated prior to reversing the mechanism of injury, has become an established orthopaedic principle. Since that time, a wealth of literature and information has appeared, aiding our understanding of the anatomy of the carpus, the biomechanics of the injury, and the surgical management of these injuries.

FIGURE 1

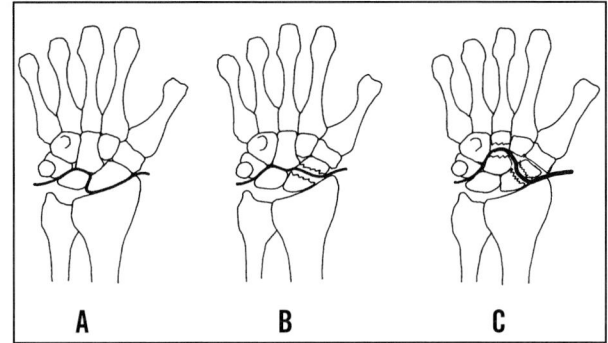

Perilunate fracture-dislocations can occur with (**A**) disruption of the scapholunate interosseous ligament (SLIL), (**B**) fracture of the scaphoid, or (**C**) fracture of the scaphoid and capitate. (Reproduced with permission from Trumble TE (ed): *Principles of Hand Surgery and Therapy*. Philadelphia, PA, WB Saunders, 2000, p 112.)

FIGURE 2

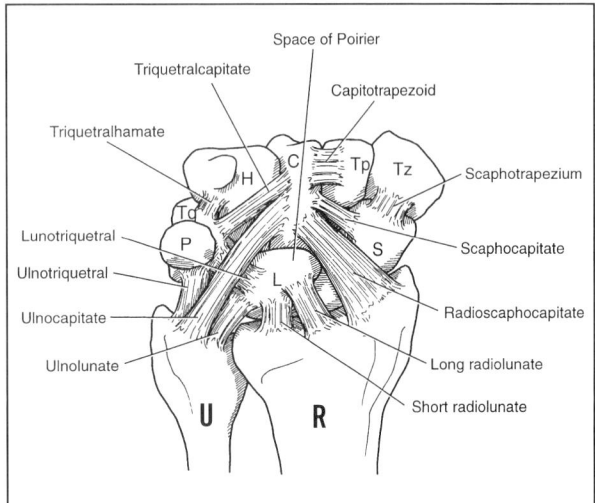

Palmar view of the ligaments of the wrist. The palmar carpal ligaments form a V-shaped pattern of support along the palmar aspect of the carpus with a weak space, known as the space of Poirier, centered at the level of the capitolunate joint. P = pisiform, Tq = triquetrum, H = hamate, C = capitate, Tp = trapezoid, Tz = trapezium, S = scaphoid, L = lunate, U = ulna, R = radius. (Reproduced with permission from Trumble TE (ed): *Principles of Hand Surgery and Therapy.* Philadelphia, PA, WB Saunders, 2000, p 92.)

FIGURE 3

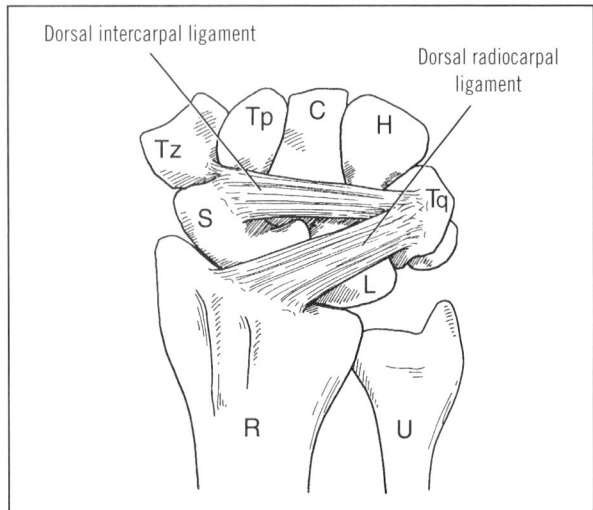

Dorsal view of the wrist. The most significant dorsal ligaments include the dorsal radiocarpal and the dorsal intercarpal ligaments. S = scaphoid, Tz = trapezium, Tp = trapezoid, C = capitate, H = hamate, Tq = triquetrum, L = lunate, R = radius, U = ulna. (Reproduced with permission from Trumble TE (ed): *Principles of Hand Surgery and Therapy.* Philadelphia, PA, WB Saunders, 2000, p 109.)

ANATOMY

The ligaments of the wrist can be divided into the intra-articular or intracapsular ligaments, including the interosseous ligaments (the scapholunate interosseous ligament [SLIL], the lunotriquetral interosseous ligament [LTIL], and the radioscapholunate ligament), the palmar capsular ligaments, and the dorsal capsular ligaments. The anatomy of the interosseous ligaments is unique in that it allows the carpal bones to rotate with respect to one another without allowing significant translation or gapping. The SLIL is one of the most important ligaments stabilizing the carpus, and it can be divided into three zones: dorsal, membranous, and palmar. The dorsal segment is the strongest and may be the most important in the causation of certain instability patterns.[2] The palmar capsular ligaments form two inverted-V–shaped patterns, creating an inverted segment that has less ligament support (the space of Poirier) (Fig. 2); the lunate dislocates through this space in lunate dislocations. The radioscaphocapitate is an important secondary stabilizer to the carpus.[3] The radioscapholunate, or ligament of Testut, was initially considered to be a key stabilizer of the carpus, but anatomic studies have demonstrated that this is a vestigial embryonic structure that serves as a vascular pedicle in the fetus. The dorsal ligaments are thinner and weaker, but they appear to play an important role in the final stages of carpal instability when static deformity occurs (Fig. 3). The dorsal intercarpal ligament appears to play the most significant role in controlling carpal motion.

PATHOMECHANICS

Carpal dislocations typically occur in young men and result from high-energy injuries. Motor vehicle accidents, falls from heights, and sports accidents are the most common causes of these injuries. The typical mechanism is believed to be hyperextension and ulnar deviation.

Mayfield and associates[4] described the sequence of events in what is called progressive perilunate instability. According to this concept, the four stages of progressive ligamentous damage occur with the wrist hyperextended and with variable degrees of ulnar deviation and forearm supination (Fig. 4). Mayfield used cadaver specimens that were tested with sudden loading to produce carpal dislocation. There was a predictable pattern of injury: the SLIL was torn, followed by a sequence of ligaments around the lunate in an ulnar direction until dislocation of the carpus occurred with or without a fracture of one of the

FIGURE 4

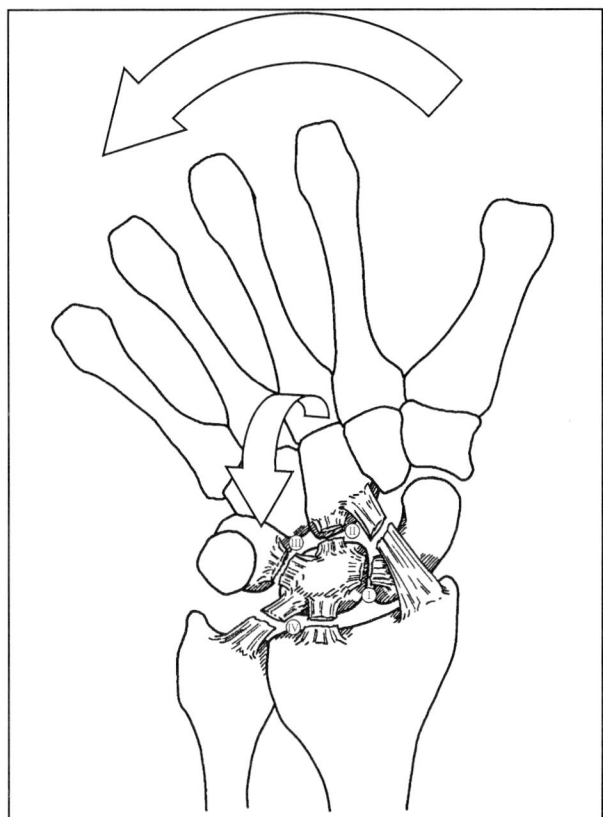

The four stages of ligament disruption that occur in the course of progressive perilunate instability, as described by Mayfield and associates. Stage I is scapholunate separation; stage II is capitolunate dislocation; stage III is triquetrolunate separation; stage IV is lunate dislocation. The large arrows demonstrate the ulnar deviation and wrist extension direction of injury. (Reproduced with permission from Trumble TE (ed): *Principles of Hand Surgery and Therapy.* Philadelphia, PA, WB Saunders, 2000, p 107.)

carpal bones.[5] The SLIL, a C-shaped intracapsular ligament, is clearly the most critical ligament in the wrist, controlling the rotation of the scaphoid and the lunate without allowing gapping or translation between the two bones. The dorsal component is the strongest segment of this crucial ligament[2] (Fig. 5).

DIAGNOSTIC IMAGING

Plain radiographs, including PA and lateral views, will show a perilunate injury, but additional views may be necessary to reveal subtle carpal fractures.[6] The lateral view is important because the dorsal displacement of the capitate with respect to the lunate is easily visualized with

FIGURE 5

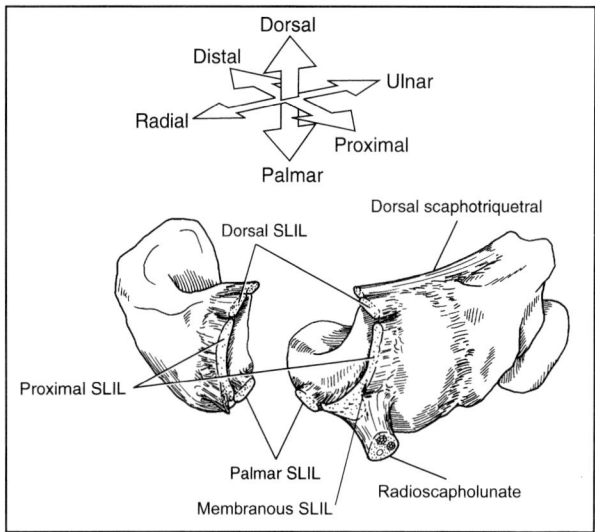

The SLIL comprises three important segments: the strong dorsal component; the thinner membranous portion, which is the weakest; and the palmar portion, which is intermediate in strength. (Reproduced with permission from Trumble TE (ed): *Principles of Hand Surgery and Therapy.* Philadelphia, PA, WB Saunders, 2000, p 92.)

FIGURE 6

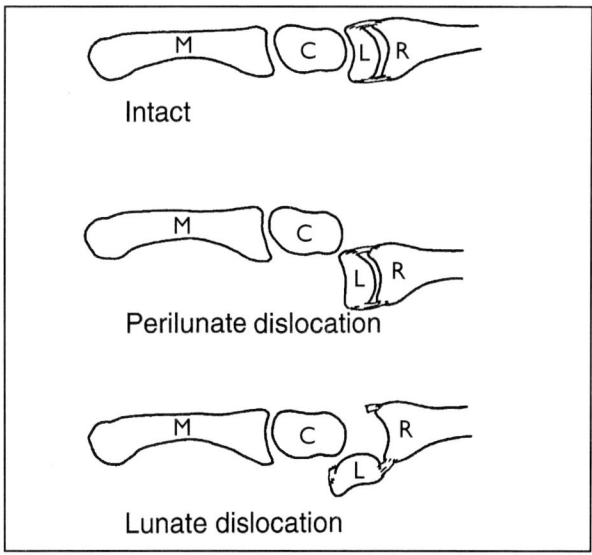

In a perilunate dislocation, the capitate is initially displaced dorsal to the lunate. In the final stages of these injuries, the capitate reduces into the fossa of the radius, displacing the lunate toward the palm. Perilunate dislocations and lunate dislocations represent either end of a spectrum of injuries caused by the same mechanism. M = metacarpal, C = capitate, L = lunate, R = radius. (Reproduced with permission from Trumble TE (ed): *Principles of Hand Surgery and Therapy.* Philadelphia, PA, WB Saunders, 2000, p 107.)

FIGURE 7

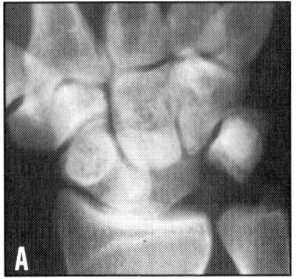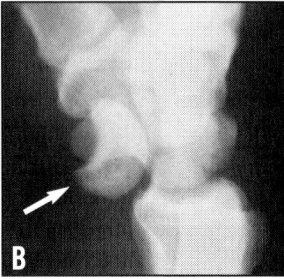

Radiographs showing a lunate dislocation. **A,** PA radiograph. **B,** On the lateral radiograph, the lunate is displaced palmarly, while the capitate articulates with the radius. (Reproduced with permission from Trumble TE (ed): *Principles of Hand Surgery and Therapy.* Philadelphia, PA, WB Saunders, 2000, p. 108.)

FIGURE 8

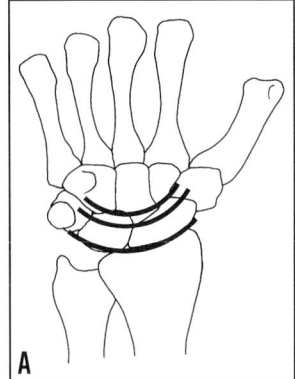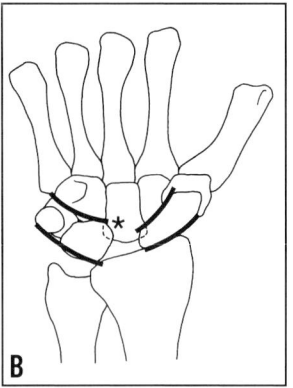

Dorsal view of the wrist. **A,** The lines of Gilula, three sets of concentric lines formed by the radial carpal and midcarpal joints, provide the basis of a good screening technique for carpal instability. **B,** Disruptions are shown in the lines of Gilula, indicating a carpal instability pattern. (Reproduced with permission from Trumble TE (ed): *Principles of Hand Surgery and Therapy.* Philadelphia, PA, WB Saunders, 2000, p 109.)

FIGURE 9

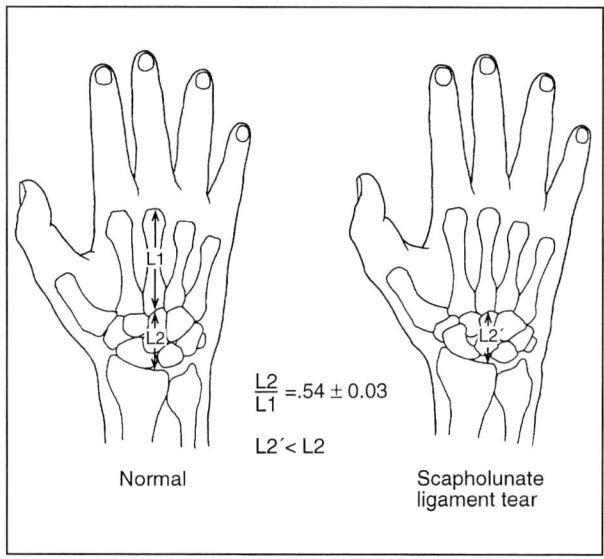

$$\frac{L2}{L1} = .54 \pm 0.03$$

$$L2' < L2$$

Normal   Scapholunate ligament tear

The normal carpal height ratio is the height of the carpus, L2, divided by the height of the third metacarpal, L1. With carpal collapse, the ratio becomes smaller as the carpal height decreases. (Reproduced with permission from Trumble TE (ed): *Principles of Hand Surgery and Therapy.* Philadelphia, PA, WB Saunders, 2000, p 91.)

injured scapholunate interval. Tomograms, nuclear scans, and three-dimensional scanning are not particularly helpful in evaluating carpal dislocations, but they may aid in localizing more subtle areas of injury, such as osteochondral fractures.

DIAGNOSIS

Perilunate injuries may be subtle both clinically and radiographically, and diagnosis is often delayed. Minami and Kaneda[8] reviewed their experience with 32 perilunate injuries and noted that only two were seen within 4 weeks of injury. In one of the largest reviews of perilunate dislocations and fracture-dislocations, the diagnosis was missed initially 25% of the time.[9] Not surprisingly, with delay, treatment becomes more difficult and outcome is adversely affected.

Clinically, pain and swelling are common, but deformity may be mild. Signs of median nerve injury may be present, and dysesthesia without motor dysfunction was noted in 16% of patients in one large series.[10] Plain PA and lateral radiographs of the wrist are almost always sufficient for diagnosis, but findings are sometimes subtle. On the PA view, the space between individual carpal bones

perilunate dislocations, and with lunate dislocations the lunate is identified within the carpal canal (Figs. 6 and 7). If the lunate or perilunate dislocations are reduced, the injury to the SLIL results in carpal instability and proximal migration of the capitate, producing breaks in the lines of Gilula[7] (Fig. 8) and a decrease in the carpal height ratio (Fig. 9). The carpal height ratio, which is the quotient of the linear distance from the distal surface of the capitate to the proximal articular surface of the scaphoid divided by the length of the third metacarpal, decreases as the capitate is driven into the proximal row through the should be uniform throughout. Uneven gapping between the carpal bones indicates disruption of their ligamentous connections. The articular surfaces of proximal and distal carpal rows should form smooth arcs at the radiocarpal and midcarpal articulations. With perilunate dislocations, these arcs are disrupted and unusual overlap of adjacent bones is seen. The normal overlap of the carpal bones seen on the lateral view can be confusing, but with careful inspection the distinctive moon shape of the lunate can be identified. In the uninjured wrist, the radius, lunate, and capitate should be relatively colinear, with the proximal convex surface of the lunate seated on the distal radius and the head of the capitate seated in the concavity of the distal lunate. In perilunate dislocations, the lunate-capitate articulation will be disrupted and the concave distal lunate will no longer articulate with the capitate. These injuries always disrupt the SLIL and may be complicated by rotatory subluxation of the scaphoid even after successful reduction. On the lateral view, the scapholunate angle should measure between 30° and 60°. With rotatory subluxation, the lunate tends to dorsiflex while the distal scaphoid flexes palmarly, causing this angle to increase.

CLASSIFICATION

Multiple classification systems have been devised to help describe carpal instability patterns and carpal fracture-dislocations. However, each emphasizes only one dimension of a problem that occurs in three dimensions. Although a complete discussion is beyond the scope of this text, a simplified but useful classification system is presented in Table 1.

TREATMENT

A full musculoskeletal examination to screen for concomitant axial or appendicular skeletal injuries is very important. Median nerve injuries can occur by direct blow as a contusion or by increased carpal canal pressures secondary to hemorrhage. In their series of 55 wrists with acute perilunate injuries, Adkison and Chapman[10] identified nine patients with median nerve dysfunction. Eight of the nine patients reported resolution of their symptoms with reduction of the carpus, but one had persistent dysesthesia, which recovered only after late carpal tunnel release. Acute median nerve deficits with injury do not require emergent nerve decompression, as the decompression may do little to change the injury. However, the patient with delayed onset of median nerve symptoms should undergo decompression of the carpal tunnel.

TABLE 1

Classification of Carpal Injuries

Injuries initiated on the radial side of the wrist (Mayfield stages I-IV)*

Mayfield stage I: SLIL tears of DISI patterns
   Class a: Partial tears; positive arthroscopy
   Class b: Partial tears; positive stress radiographs
   Class c: Complete tears; positive static radiographs with gapping between scaphoid and lunate or scapholunate angle > 60°
   Class d: Complete SLIL tear with degenerative changes
Mayfield stages II-IV: Carpal dislocation with or without fractures
   Perilunate dislocations (palmar and dorsal)
      Lunate dislocation
      Transscaphoid perilunate dislocations
      Transscaphoid, transcapitate perilunate dislocations
      Perilunate fracture-dislocations involving the triquetrum

Ulnar, midcarpal, or VISI patterns

Vertical shear injuries of the carpus

*Mayfield's stages of progressive perilunate instability are shown in Fig. 4.

Surgery is the definitive treatment of these complex injuries. Adkison and Chapman[10] reviewed a large number of acute perilunate injuries and found that loss of reduction occurred in 59% of wrists where initial anatomic closed reduction was achieved and a cast was applied. Apergis and associates[11] compared the outcomes of eight perilunate injuries treated with closed reduction and casting to the outcomes for 20 patients treated with open reduction and internal fixation. The clinical outcome was fair or poor in all patients treated with casting alone, while 65% of those treated with open reduction and internal fixation had good or excellent results. The authors also concluded that these injuries are too unstable to be treated without fixation. Even though surgery is recommended, a closed reduction should be performed if the surgery is delayed for any reason. Often the patient will have sustained other severe injuries that will take priority.

In nearly all of these dislocations, the capitate is displaced dorsally. The carpus should be reduced as soon as

FIGURE 10

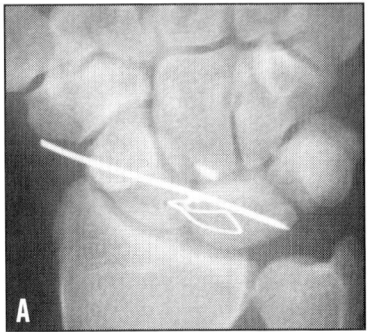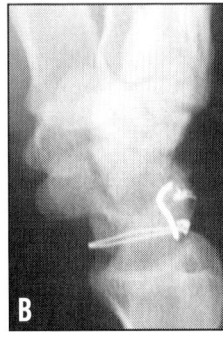

Radiographs of a perilunate dislocation repaired by open reduction and internal fixation through a dorsal approach. **A**, PA radiograph showing the SLIL secured with a cerclage wire in addition to K-wires. Suture anchors are used to reattach portions of the SLIL to the lunate. **B**, Lateral radiograph demonstrating the correct alignment of the lunate with the capitate. (Reproduced with permission from Trumble TE (ed): *Principles of Hand Surgery and Therapy*. Philadelphia, PA, WB Saunders, 2000, p 113.)

FIGURE 11

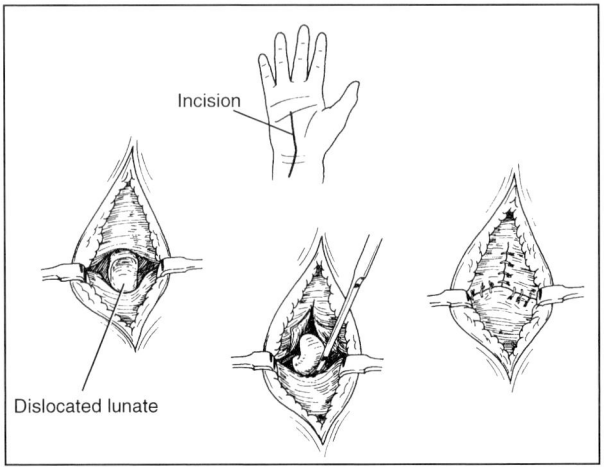

The extended carpal tunnel approach. (Reproduced with permission from Trumble TE (ed): *Principles of Hand Surgery and Therapy*. Philadelphia, PA, WB Saunders, 2000, p 114.)

possible by extending the wrist to recreate the deformity and applying dorsal pressure to reduce the capitate into the lunate fossa. Open reduction and repair of the SLIL and lunotriquetral ligaments is indicated in all perilunate and lunate dislocations. For the initial surgical approach, a dorsal longitudinal incision centered on the wrist is recommended. The third dorsal compartment is released, and the extensor pollicus longus (EPL) is retracted radially. The fourth compartment is sharply elevated off the dorsal capsule, and a longitudinal capsulotomy is made to expose the ruptured SLIL and LTIL as well as to reduce the scaphoid to the lunate and the lunate to the triquetrum. The SLIL is usually avulsed off bone rather than as a midsubstance tear. The ligament avulsions can be repaired with suture anchors. The LTIL can be repaired by passing the sutures through bone tunnels or with a suture anchor. The suture anchors dramatically increase the accuracy and strength of the repairs compared to bone tunnels. Intraoperative fluoroscopy is essential to correctly align the scaphoid to the lunate. Frequently, a Kirschner wire (K-wire) is placed vertically into the scaphoid to use as a "joystick" to correct the palmar rotation of the scaphoid. The direct appearance of the scapholunate articulation can be deceptive, and it is important to check intraoperative fluoroscopy to ensure that the correct alignment is achieved. In addition to repairing the SLIL and LTIL, additional internal fixation to stabilize the carpus is required. Two K-wires pinning the scaphoid to the lunate and two K-wires pinning the triquetrum to the lunate

can be used, but pins from the carpus to the radius are avoided. We prefer an intraosseous wiring technique that Almquist and associates[12] initially used for chronic ligament reconstruction. A separate palmar approach is necessary, similar to that described later for lunate dislocations. The cannula of a 14-gauge intravenous catheter is drilled through the proximal pole of the scaphoid, and a 22-gauge catheter is passed from dorsal to palmar through the cannula. The cannula is then removed and drilled through the lunate so that the wire can be passed from palmar to dorsal through the lunate. The next sequence of steps is placing the suture anchors, followed by tightening the wire and finally, tying the sutures attached to the anchors. This approach does require a second incision, but it avoids the placement of scapholunate K-wires, which can be very irritating, and it allows earlier wrist motion. With the intraosseous wire, wrist flexion can be started in 6 weeks, as compared with 12 weeks with K-wires. The wrist is immobilized for 6 to 8 weeks before starting range-of-motion exercises with a removable splint. The cerclage wire usually breaks as wrist motion is regained, but it rarely requires removal[12] (Fig. 10).

Most authors recommend ligament repair at the time of open reduction. Palmer and associates[13] compared outcomes in four patients treated with open reduction, pin fixation, and ligament repair with outcomes in six patients who underwent closed reduction and percutaneous pin fixation without ligament repair. Patients who did not undergo ligament repair did as well as those who did,

FIGURE 12

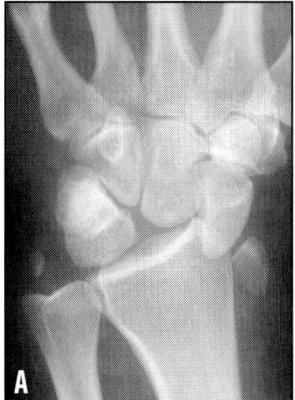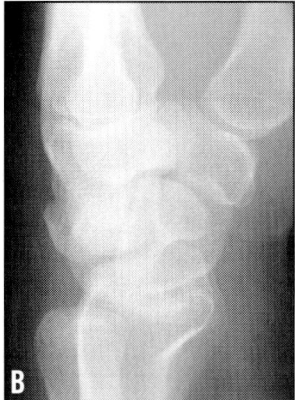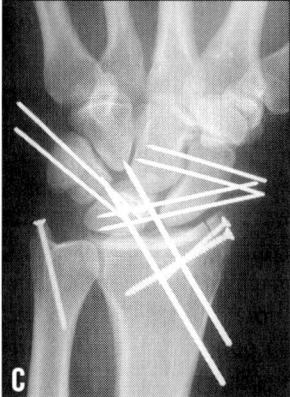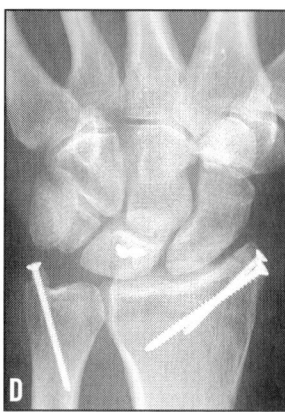

Perilunate dislocations involving fractures of the radial and ulnar styloids. **A,** PA radiograph of a perilunate dislocation involving fractures of the radial and ulnar styloids. **B,** Lateral radiograph showing the dorsal dislocation of the capitate in the perilunate dislocation shown in A; the fractures of the radial styloid and ulnar styloid cannot be seen. **C,** Radiograph of a highly unstable perilunate dislocation that required internal fixation of both styloids in addition to pinning across the midcarpal and radial carpal joints as well as repair of the SLIL with suture anchors. **D,** PA radiograph showing the proper alignment of the scaphoid and lunate after removing the K-wires. (Reproduced with permission from Trumble TE (ed): *Principles of Hand Surgery and Therapy.* Philadelphia, PA, WB Saunders, 2000, p 117.)

although intercarpal relations were maintained more consistently in the repaired group. Minami and Kaneda[8] compared results in 12 patients who underwent open reduction and interosseous ligament repair with 20 patients in whom open reduction and pin fixation was performed without ligament repair. At an average follow-up of 5 years, they found that repair or reconstruction of the dorsal SLIL improved clinical results and reduced the incidence of carpal instability.

Palmarly displaced lunocapitate dislocations are rare, representing less than 3% of all perilunate injuries.[14] Open reduction using both palmar and dorsal approaches and internal fixation with wires or screws is the method of choice. The combined approach also produces favorable outcomes for the more commonly encountered dorsal perilunate dislocations.[15]

The treatment of lunate dislocations is similar to that for perilunate dislocations except that a separate palmar approach may be needed to reduce the lunate. Occasionally, the lunate can be successfully reduced by (1) flexing the wrist to remove tension from the palmar ligaments, (2) applying palmar pressure over the lunate followed by wrist extension to reduce the lunate into its fossa on the radius, and (3) flexing the wrist to reduce the capitate into the lunate. If the lunate can be reduced by manipulation, a dorsal approach, as described for perilunate dislocations, will suffice unless the cerclage wiring technique is chosen. If the lunate cannot be reduced by closed methods, an

extended carpal tunnel approach will expose the dislocated lunate and facilitate reduction of the lunate and repair of the palmar ligaments (Fig. 11). When fractures of the radial styloid or ulnar styloid accompany the perilunate dislocation, internal fixation is advised because the ligament attachments to these fragments provide essential support of the wrist (Fig. 12).

DELAYED TREATMENT

Delayed presentation or diagnosis is not uncommon with these injuries. While some untreated patients report minimal symptoms, long-term follow-up suggests the outcome is typically poor. Pain, weakness, and loss of motion are common, with posttraumatic arthrosis, carpal tunnel syndrome, and attritional flexor tendon rupture reported. One of the largest studies of perilunate injuries reported on 15 patients who were untreated for an average of 22 years.[9] These patients had worse clinical scores than those treated by any method shortly following injury. Because of this relatively dismal natural history, surgery should be considered regardless of the length of time since injury.

Late treatment options include open reduction and internal fixation, lunate excision, proximal row carpectomy, and wrist fusion. Few series have compared these different approaches. Seigert and associates[16] reviewed a series of 15 patients with perilunate injuries treated an average of 17 weeks after injury (minimum 6 weeks) with a mean follow-up of 6 years. Open reduction and internal fixation was performed in six patients, carpal bone excision in four, proximal row carpectomy in two, wrist arthrodesis in two, and carpal tunnel release in one. Keeping in mind the small number of patients involved, the results were as follows: Open reduction and internal fixation provided the most reliable improvement. Although proximal row carpectomy and wrist fusion also produced significant improvement, the level of improvement did not exceed that of open reduction. In the patient troubled only by symptoms of carpal tunnel syndrome, simple release provided expected relief. Patients treated with carpal bone excision alone did uniformly poorly.

Inoue and Shionoya[17] reviewed 28 patients with perilunate injuries treated at least 6 weeks following injury. Proximal row carpectomy was performed in 16 patients, open reduction and internal fixation in six, lunate excision in four, and carpal tunnel release with partial lunate excision in two. At a mean follow-up of 6 years, clinical results were best overall in patients treated with open reduction and internal fixation. Proximal row carpectomy appeared to be a reasonable option in patients without damage to the articular surface of the capitate. The authors also concluded that lunate excision alone was a poor treatment option.

Open reduction should be considered, even if the injury occurred long ago. Although open reduction becomes progressively more difficult over time, there is no time limit after which it should be ruled out. Reduction offers the greatest potential for restoring more normal wrist biomechanics and preserves both proximal row carpectomy and wrist fusion as treatment options. Proximal row carpectomy is a reasonable option if reduction cannot be achieved and the head of the capitate has not been significantly injured. Arthrodesis is also effective in relieving pain and improving strength.

Outcomes

The outcome for untreated perilunate injuries is generally poor. In a multicenter review, Herzberg and associates[9] identified 15 patients who were untreated for an average of 22 years following injury. Motion and grip strength were poor; pain and activity restriction were less common. Posttraumatic arthrosis was uniformly present, and carpal tunnel syndrome was common. The high rate of delayed presentation and diagnosis in this and other series, however, indicates that many patients have minimal symptoms. In reviewing the outcome of 115 perilunate injuries with a mean 6-year follow-up, the authors noted that although the pattern of injury had little influence on outcome, open injury and delay in treatment did adversely affect results. Good radiographic outcome tended to correlate with good clinical outcome, but many poor radiographic outcomes were also well tolerated. The best results were achieved with open reduction and internal fixation.

Sotereanos and associates[18] reviewed the outcome of 11 perilunate injuries treated at one institution with a uniform approach. Patients were treated with open reduction and internal fixation using combined dorsal and palmar approaches at an average of 13 hours after injury. Maximal recovery of motion and strength typically occurred between 12 and 18 months. At a mean follow-up of 30 months, wrist flexion and extension averaged 71% of that of the unaffected wrist. Radial-ulnar deviation averaged 70%, grip strength 77%, lateral pinch 84%, and tip pinch 78%. Radiographically, no significant carpal instability was detected, although posttraumatic arthrosis developed in two patients. Nine of 11 patients reported high satisfaction with the outcome.

Summary

Perilunate injuries severely disrupt normal wrist function and are prone to poor clinical outcomes if untreated. Early diagnosis, accurate reduction, and stable internal fixation improve outcomes. Even when presentation is delayed, surgery should be considered to maximize recovery of function. Closed reduction often achieves gross realignment of the wrist, but accurate reduction of the small irregular carpal articulations generally requires open reduction. A dorsal approach provides the best view of these small joints, but a palmar approach may be necessary as well. K-wires inserted into the carpal bones to allow direct manipulation facilitate accurate reduction. These injuries are highly unstable and always require temporary pin or wire fixation to reliably maintain reduction after ligament repair. Ligament repair at the time of reduction has not been shown conclusively to improve outcome, but it appears to minimize the risk of resulting carpal instability. Pins are typically removed after 6 to 8 weeks, but final recovery of motion and strength often takes 12 to 18 months.

REFERENCES

1. The classic: Injuries of the wrist: A radiological study. By Etienne Destot. 1926. *Clin Orthop* 1986;202:3-11.

2. Berger RA: The gross and histologic anatomy of the scapholunate interosseous ligament. *J Hand Surg Am* 1996;21:170-178.

3. Weaver L, Tencer AF, Trumble TE: Tensions in the palmar ligaments of the wrist: I. The normal wrist. *J Hand Surg Am* 1994;19:464-474.

4. Mayfield JK, Johnson RP, Kilcoyne RK: Carpal dislocations: Pathomechanics and progressive perilunar instability. *J Hand Surg Am* 1980;5:226-241.

5. Mayfield JK: Wrist ligamentous anatomy and pathogenesis of carpal instability. *Orthop Clin North Am* 1984;15:209-216.

6. Kozin SH: Perilunate injuries: Diagnosis and treatment. *J Am Acad Orthop Surg* 1998;6:114-120.

7. Gilula LA: Carpal injuries: Analytic approach and case exercises. *AJR Am J Roentgenol* 1979;133:503-517.

8. Minami A, Kaneda K: Repair and/or reconstruction of scapholunate interosseous ligament in lunate and perilunate dislocations. *J Hand Surg Am* 1993;18:1099-1106.

9. Herzberg G, Comtet JJ, Linscheid RL, Amadio PC, Cooney WP, Stalder J: Perilunate dislocations and fracture-dislocations: A multicenter study. *J Hand Surg Am* 1993;18:768-779.

10. Adkison JW, Chapman MW: Treatment of acute lunate and perilunate dislocations. *Clin Orthop* 1982;164:199-207.

11. Apergis E, Maris J, Theodoratos G, Pavlakis D, Antoniou N: Perilunate dislocations and fracture-dislocations: Closed and early open reduction compared in 28 cases. *Acta Orthop Scand Suppl* 1997;275:55-59.

12. Almquist EE, Bach AW, Sack JT, Fuhs SE, Newman DM: Four-bone ligament reconstruction for treatment of chronic complete scapholunate separation. *J Hand Surg Am* 1991;16:322-327.

13. Palmer AK, Dobyns JH, Linscheid RL: Management of post-traumatic instability of the wrist secondary to ligament rupture. *J Hand Surg Am* 1978;3:507-532.

14. Israeli A, Engel J, Ganel A: Recurrent volar carpal perilunate subluxation. *Arch Orthop Trauma Surg* 1982;99:285-286.

15. Melone CP Jr, Murphy MS, Raskin KB: Perilunate injuries: Repair by dual dorsal and volar approaches. *Hand Clin* 2000;16:439-448.

16. Siegert JJ, Frassica FJ, Amadio PC: Treatment of chronic perilunate dislocations. *J Hand Surg Am* 1988;13:206-212.

17. Inoue G, Shionoya K: Late treatment of unreduced perilunate dislocations. *J Hand Surg Br* 1999;24:221-225.

18. Sotereanos DG, Mitsionis GJ, Giannakopoulos PN, Tomaino MM, Herndon JH: Perilunate dislocation and fracture dislocation: A critical analysis of the volar-dorsal approach. *J Hand Surg Am* 1997;22:49-56.

CHAPTER 5

SCAPHOLUNATE INSTABILITY

CHRISTOPHER H. ALLAN, MD
THOMAS E. TRUMBLE, MD

The scapholunate interosseous ligament (SLIL) is a three-sided structure joining the scaphoid and lunate bones of the carpus. The proximal portion of the ligament is actually a thin fibrocartilaginous membrane that does not contribute significantly to the stability of the scapholunate articulation. The palmar and particularly the dorsal aspects of the SLIL are stronger and are responsible for ensuring linkage between the scaphoid and the lunate during wrist motion.[1]

The significance of the SLIL lies in the importance of linking the motion of the scaphoid and lunate bones. The scaphoid, the lunate, and the triquetrum are joined by strong interosseous ligaments that cause these bones—the proximal row of the carpus—to move as a unit. The scaphoid sits in an irregular fossa at the end of the radius and flexes with radial deviation as it is compressed between the radius and the trapezium. When the interosseous ligaments of the proximal row are intact, the entire proximal row follows the scaphoid into flexion (Fig. 1). Similarly, in ulnar deviation, the triquetrum is forced into extension by sliding down its helicoid joint with the hamate, and the rest of the proximal row extends with it[2] (Fig. 2). The proximal row also flexes with pure wrist flexion and extends with wrist extension, although motion occurs at the midcarpal joint as well.

An injury to the SLIL can disrupt these linked motions, resulting in independent motion of the scaphoid with respect to the lunate and triquetrum. The scaphoid still flexes with wrist flexion and radial deviation—more so, in fact, because the tendency of the triquetrohamate joint to extend the proximal row, which exerts a counterbalancing effect, is no longer transmitted to the scaphoid. For the same reason, the scaphoid no longer extends with wrist extension or ulnar deviation. The lunate follows the triquetrum into extension, no longer balanced with flex-

ion forces through an attachment to the scaphoid. These changes in position may be apparent only with motion or loading with gripping activities, in which case the instability is termed dynamic, or they may be present at rest, in which case the instability is termed static.

In acute SLIL disruption, the changes described here can cause radial-sided wrist pain. The patient experiences sudden, uncomfortable, abnormally increased motion of the scaphoid, often referred to as a "clunk." Over time, the scaphoid can develop a fixed flexion posture, where it is no longer seated in the radial fossa, and the radioscaphoid joint cartilage can erode with repetitive motion of the wrist through the incongruent joint. This occurs first at the radial styloid/scaphoid interface and then progresses to involve the entire radioscaphoid joint. The lunate can adopt a position of fixed extension, although its rounded proximal surface will still articulate smoothly with the rounded lunate fossa of the distal radius; therefore, arth-

FIGURE 1

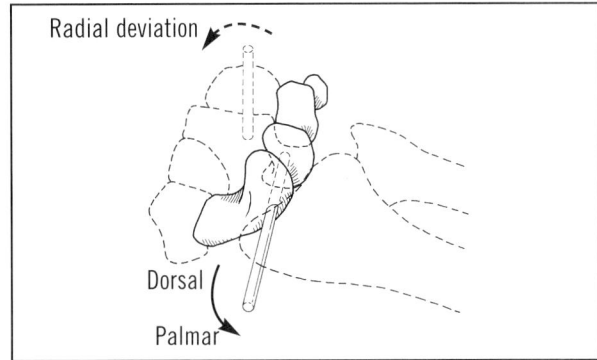

With radial deviation, the articular contacts force the scaphoid to rotate into flexion. The scaphoid transmits rotational force to the lunate and triquetrum via the SLIL. (Reproduced with permission from Trumble TE (ed): *Principles of Hand Surgery and Therapy*. Philadelphia, PA, WB Saunders, 2000, p 91.)

FIGURE 2

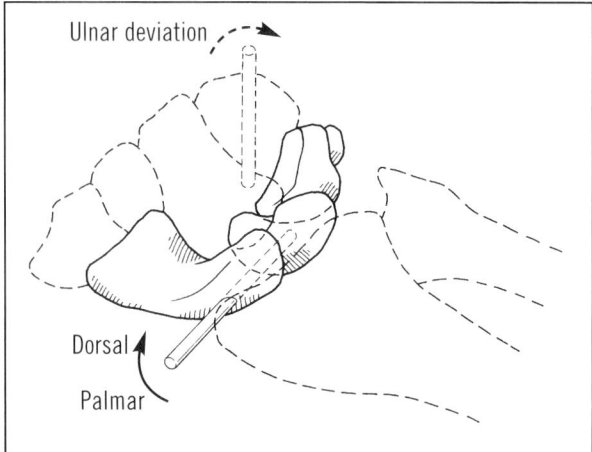

With ulnar deviation, the helicoid contact between the triquetrum and hamate causes the triquetrum to rotate into extension. The triquetrum causes the lunate to rotate dorsally because of the lunotriquetral interosseous ligament (LTIL), and the scaphoid extends or rotates dorsally because of the SLIL. (Reproduced with permission from Trumble TE (ed): *Principles of Hand Surgery and Therapy*. Philadelphia, PA, WB Saunders, 2000, p 90.)

ritic changes in the radiolunate joint as a result of SLIL injury are rare. In the final stage of arthritic degeneration, the capitate migrates proximally into the gap between the fixed, rotated scaphoid and the lunate, eroding the cartilage of the capitolunate joint.[3] To summarize, acute disruption of the SLIL can lead to painful instability, which can progress to chronic degenerative arthritis.

INJURY PATTERNS

Much of the current understanding of the mechanism of injury to the SLIL comes from work done by Mayfield and associates,[4] who described a reproducible pattern of carpal bone or ligament failure occurring in a progressive fashion (see chapter 2). The injury mechanism associated with this pattern of ligament failure typically leads to wrist extension, ulnar deviation, and intercarpal supination, with structures failing beginning on the radial side of the wrist. The level of energy of the injury determines the extent of disruption of wrist structures. This pattern of injury has been called progressive perilunate injury because the structures fail in a sequence progressing from radial to ulnar around the lunate. The injury begins with fracture of the radial styloid, fracture of the scaphoid, tearing of the SLIL, or some combination of these. Injuries of greater energy traverse the capitolunate

joint, occasionally fracturing the capitate, and progress through the lunotriquetral interosseous ligament (LTIL) or the triquetrum. As injury forces progress ulnarly, the ulnar styloid may be fractured, or the triangular fibrocartilage complex (TFCC) may be disrupted. In its most severe form, the injury results in dislocation (usually palmar) of the lunate. Within the broad spectrum of perilunate instabilities, SLIL injuries can be considered a Mayfield stage I perilunate injury.

PATIENT EVALUATION

History

Patients with acute injuries of the SLIL generally recall a recent injury, often a fall on an outstretched arm, with a sudden onset of radial-sided wrist pain followed by varying degrees of discomfort with wrist motion. Chronic SLIL injuries sometimes present quite late, and often the patient will not recall a specific injury.

Physical Examination

Swelling of the dorsoradial aspect of the wrist may be evident. Pain may limit motion, particularly radial deviation, and tenderness over the SLIL (approximately 1 cm distal to Lister's tubercle) may be present. The scaphoid shift test may reveal scaphoid instability. In this test, the examiner locates the palmar prominence of the distal pole of the scaphoid (most easily identified when the wrist is in radial deviation) and applies dorsally directed pressure to the distal pole while moving the wrist from ulnar to radial deviation and back (Fig. 3). An intact SLIL will keep the scaphoid seated in the scaphoid fossa of the distal radius, but an incompetent ligament will allow dorsal subluxation of the scaphoid proximal pole over the dorsal lip of the radius with progressive radial deviation (Fig. 4). Returning the wrist to an ulnarly deviated position allows for reduction of the subluxation; the subluxation and reduction generally cause pain and a palpable clunk.[5] The test must be repeated on the uninjured side for comparison because ligamentous laxity can lead to a positive test without injury being present. For patients with incomplete tears of the SLIL, this test will often be painful without producing the characteristic clunk.

Imaging Studies

Initial radiographs should include neutral PA, neutral lateral, grip PA, and ulnar deviation PA views. Comparison views of the contralateral wrist may be useful when the diagnosis is uncertain. In patients with static SLIL insta-

FIGURE 3

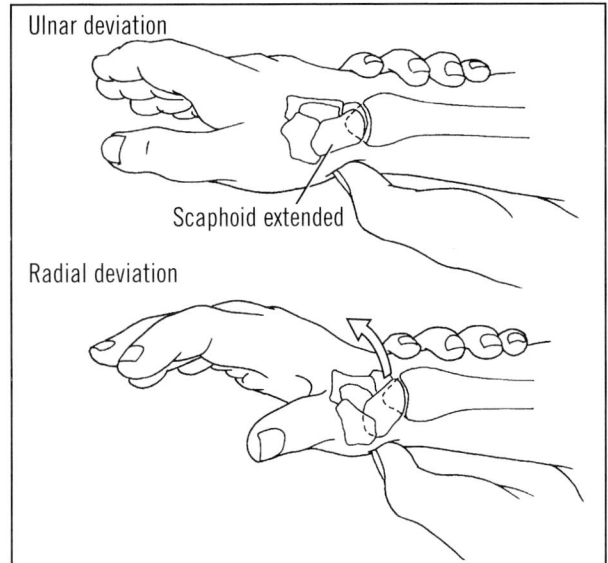

The scaphoid shift test is performed by placing pressure on the scaphoid tubercle and moving the wrist from ulnar deviation to radial deviation. (Reproduced with permission from Trumble TE (ed): *Principles of Hand Surgery and Therapy*. Philadelphia, PA, WB Saunders, 2000, p 107.)

FIGURE 4

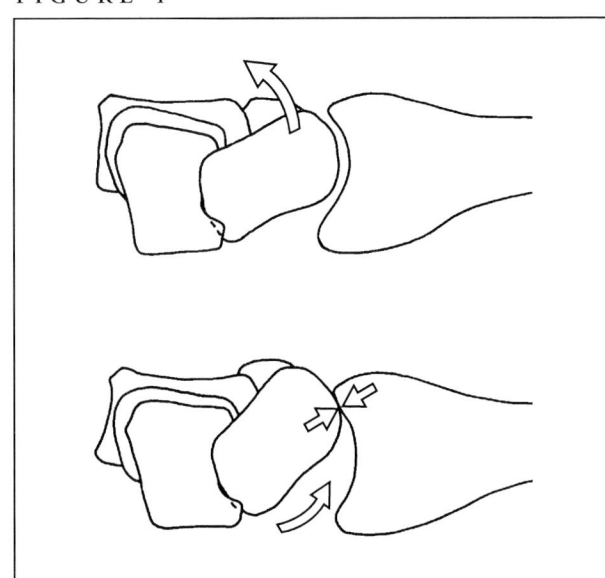

When the SLIL is incompetent, the scaphoid shift test causes dorsal translation of the scaphoid, producing a clunk as the proximal pole is forced into the dorsal rim of the radius. (Reproduced with permission from Trumble TE (ed): *Principles of Hand Surgery and Therapy*. Philadelphia, PA, WB Saunders, 2000, p 108.)

FIGURE 5

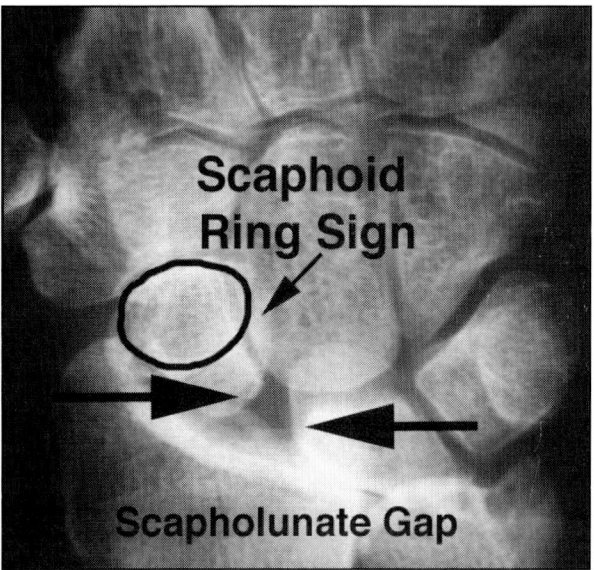

PA radiograph showing the "ring sign" and a widened scapholunate gap. (Reproduced with permission from Trumble TE (ed): *Principles of Hand Surgery and Therapy*. Philadelphia, PA, WB Saunders, 2000, p 108.)

bility, the PA views may show the following: widening of the scapholunate gap (maximized in the grip and ulnar deviation PA views); shortening of the flexed scaphoid, resulting in the cortical "ring sign" as the proximal and distal poles overlie one another; and, in late cases, arthritic changes (Fig. 5). Watson and Ballet[3] organized the latter finding into a three-part classification termed the scapholunate advanced collapse (SLAC) pattern (Fig. 6). The lateral view may show an increased scapholunate angle, which is the angle formed by the long axes of the scaphoid and the lunate (Fig. 7). This angle normally ranges from 30° to 60°, with an average of 47°.[6] After SLIL disruption, however, the scapholunate angle can approach 90°, as the now-unlinked scaphoid flexes and the lunate and triquetrum tilt into extension. An SLIL injury should be suspected in any patient who has a scapholunate angle greater than 60° and an appropriate history and positive findings on physical examination.

Many additional radiographic views have been described in an effort to detect abnormal motion of the scaphoid and lunate. Other imaging techniques used to detect static instability include arthrography, bone scintigraphy, and MRI. Arthrography documents communicating defects, but these may not represent functionally significant tears.[7] Bone scintigraphy has been reported as highly sensitive

FIGURE 6

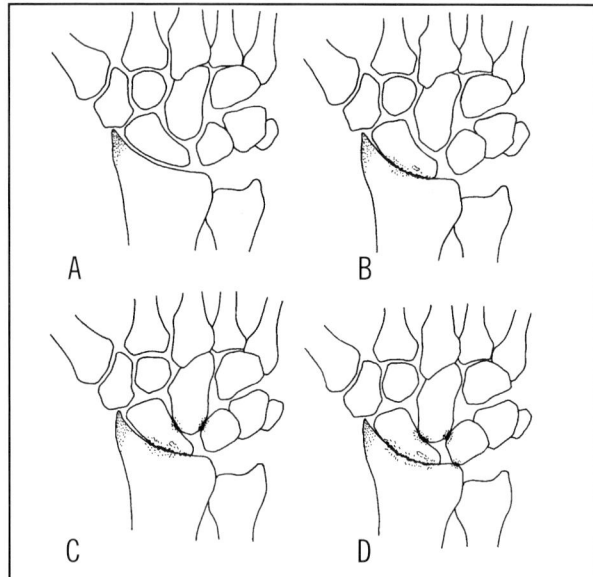

Stages of the SLAC pattern. **A**, Stage 1 is characterized by beaking of the radial styloid and narrowing of its articulation with the scaphoid. **B**, In stage 2, narrowing of the entire radioscaphoid joint is evident. **C**, In stage 3, proximal migration of the capitate occurs, leading to capitolunate joint degeneration. **D** In stage 4, degeneration of the radiolunate joint occurs. (Reproduced with permission from Trumble TE (ed): *Principles of Hand Surgery and Therapy.* Philadelphia, PA, WB Saunders, 2000, p 406.)

FIGURE 7

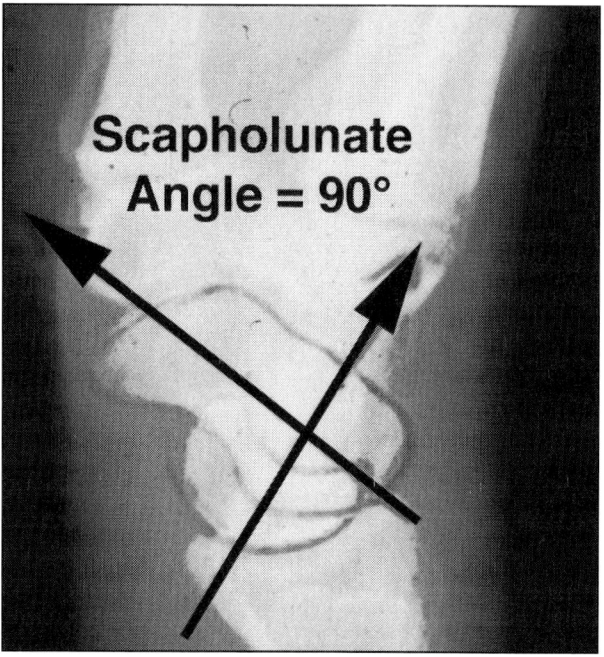

Lateral view showing increased scapholunate angle. (Reproduced with permission from Trumble TE (ed): *Principles of Hand Surgery and Therapy.* Philadelphia, PA, WB Saunders, 2000, p 108.)

(~98%) for complete tears but much less so for partial ligament injuries.[8] MRI has been used successfully to evaluate TFCC injuries but has a reported sensitivity of only 37% for SLIL tears.[9] Cineradiography is unique among these studies in its ability to allow evaluation of dynamic instability; a simple alternative is to have the patient move the wrist through a range of motion under an office Fluoroscan device (Fluoroscan Imaging Systems, Bedford, MA).

Finally, arthroscopy has become widely used in the evaluation of patients with wrist pain and suspected SLIL injuries, in part because of the limitations of the imaging studies just described. The most accurate diagnostic technique, arthroscopy, is also the most invasive. A classification of ligament injuries based on arthroscopic appearance and examination has been devised by Geissler and associates[10] (Fig. 8). Dynamic instability can be difficult to detect, even with arthroscopy. No perfect imaging study exists; all of the studies described must be used in conjunction with a careful history and examination.

CLASSIFICATION

The decisions whether to pursue surgical intervention for an SLIL injury and, if so, whether primary repair of the SLIL is possible, are the most important in patient management. The first step in the decision-making process is to classify the injury; injuries can be classified as either stable or unstable and either acute or chronic. Stable injuries may include partial tears of the SLIL with associated pain and swelling, occasionally with ganglion formation, but without findings of instability on radiographic or physical examination as described earlier. Unstable injuries can be either static or dynamic, that is, with or without radiographic findings of abnormal carpal alignment on plain radiographs or on stress or "fist" radiographs. Clinicians differ in defining the time period during which an injury may be considered acute, but it is generally considered to extend for 8 to 12 weeks from the time of injury. After this time, the injury is often considered chronic. Nevertheless, Lavernia and associates[11] reported encountering a surgically repairable ligament as

FIGURE 8

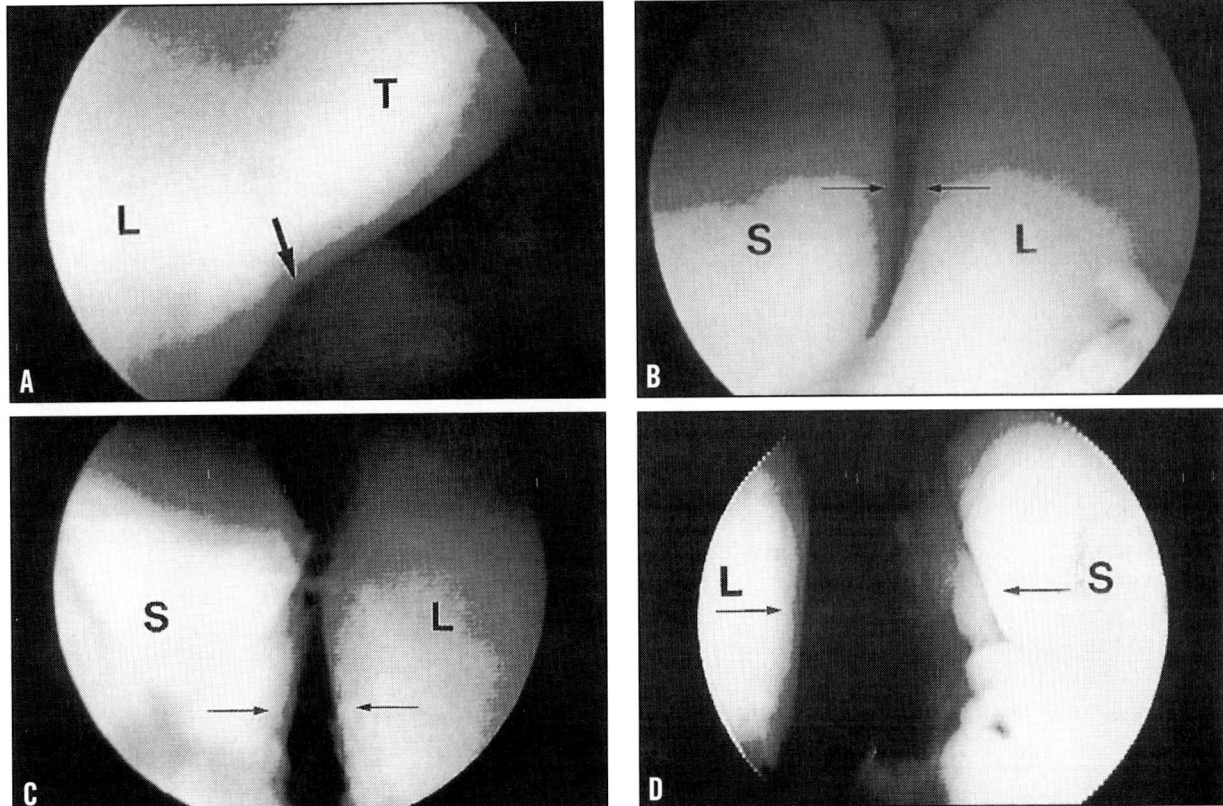

Grades of ligament injury according to the classification by Geissler and associates. **A,** Arthroscopic view of the normal concave appearance between the carpal bones as seen from the radiocarpal space (arrow). There are no separations or step-offs. L = lunate, T = triquetrum. **B,** Arthroscopic view of a grade II tear of an interosseous ligament, showing loss of the normal congruent appearance of the carpal bones. There is a step-off between the scaphoid and the lunate, as seen from the midcarpal space (arrows). S = scaphoid **C,** Arthroscopic view of a grade III tear of an interosseous ligament. There is a gap between the scaphoid and the lunate, as seen from the midcarpal space (arrows). A similar gap between the carpal bones is seen from the radiocarpal space, and a probe can be passed between the carpal bones. **D,** Arthroscopic view of a grade IV tear of an interosseous ligament. There is a larger separation between the carpal bones, as seen from the midcarpal space (arrows). A 2.7-mm arthroscope can pass between the carpal bones from the midcarpal space to the radiocarpal space. (Reproduced with permission from Geissler WB, Freeland AE, Savoie FH, McIntyre LW, Whipple TL: Intracarpal soft-tissue lesions associated with an intra-articular fracture of the distal end of the radius. *J Bone Joint Surg Am* 1996;78:357-365.)

late as 7 years after an injury, so the classification of an injury as either acute or chronic can be arbitrary. The surgeon must therefore be prepared for several possibilities when surgical treatment is planned. Acute injuries typically have a better prognosis because the potential to maintain scapholunate alignment following repair is improved.

Further classification of chronic injuries includes determining the reducibility of the scaphoid flexion deformity and the presence and degree of osteoarthritic changes. These determinations often can be made only during surgery.

Trumble's[12] subclassification of the Mayfield type I SLIL injuries separates the injuries into the following categories: Ia: symptoms present, but radiographic studies negative; Ib: arthrogram or arthroscopy positive, but no evidence of static or dynamic instability; Ic: dynamic instability present; and Id: static instability present.

TREATMENT

Stable Injuries

For patients with stable injuries (types Ia and Ib: no instability on radiographs or physical examination), a short

FIGURE 9

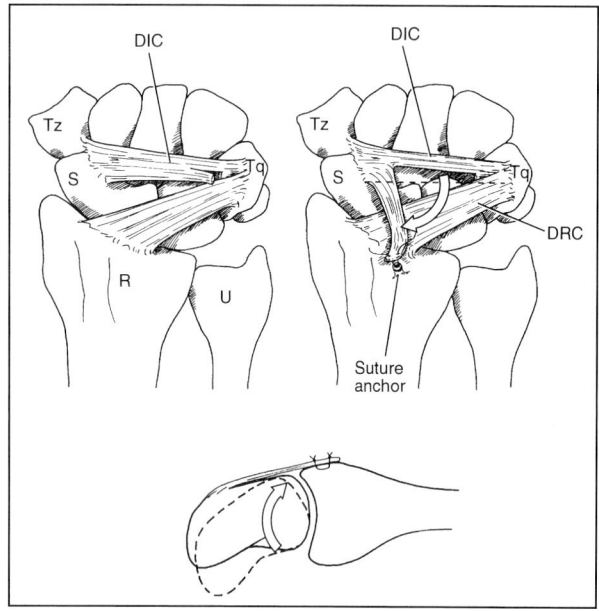

In a modification of the Blatt procedure, Berger[1,2] described rotating a portion of the DIC ligament and securing it to the distal radius. Tz = trapezium, S = scaphoid, Tq = triquetrum, R = radius, U = ulna. (Reproduced with permission from Trumble TE (ed): *Principles of Hand Surgery and Therapy.* Philadelphia, PA, WB Saunders, 2000, p 109.)

FIGURE 10

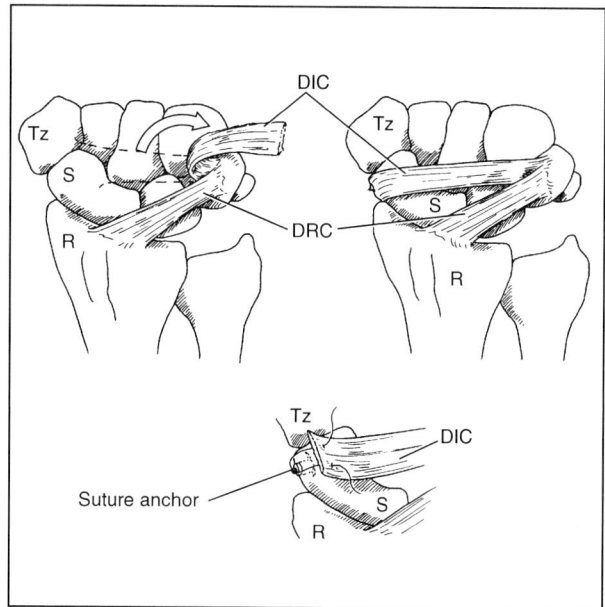

The capsulodesis described by Slater and associates involves the advancement of a portion of the DIC ligament to a point along the radial surface of the scaphoid. Tz = trapezium, S = scaphoid, R = radius. (Reproduced with permission from Trumble TE (ed): *Principles of Hand Surgery and Therapy.* Philadelphia, PA, WB Saunders, 2000, p 110.)

course of cast or splint immobilization with early follow-up may be very helpful. If the diagnosis is at all uncertain, additional imaging studies are indicated because a missed acute injury can become chronic, with fewer treatment options available. Patients should return in 2 weeks for follow-up examination and radiographs. Because partial SLIL injuries can result in the formation of occasionally painful ganglia, which may take several months to become evident, even these stable injuries warrant follow-up for some time. Patients should be advised to modify their activities long-term to avoiding loading the wrist in extension.

Acute Injuries With Dynamic and Static Instability and Chronic Injuries With Dynamic Instability

Acute unstable injuries and symptomatic patients with dynamic instability require surgery. If the SLIL is repairable, the scaphoid is reducible from its flexed posture, and there are no arthritic changes, most authors now recommend primary repair of the ligament using either drill holes or suture anchors, augmented with some type of

dorsal capsulodesis.[11] The SLIL can be reinforced using the dorsal capsule or a portion of the dorsal retinaculum (dorsal capsulodesis) as described by Blatt[13] and since modified by others.[1,2,14] This procedure theoretically provides a checkrein that decreases palmar flexion of the scaphoid and prevents the scaphoid from shifting dorsally.

Capsulodesis Techniques

Blatt Procedure The original procedure as described by Blatt[13] involves advancement of the dorsal wrist capsule to the distal pole of the scaphoid in order to permanently reduce the palmar flexion of the scaphoid. Exposure for this procedure is performed through a dorsal midline approach. The third dorsal compartment is released, and the extensor pollicis longus is retracted radially. The fourth dorsal compartment is carefully dissected off the dorsal capsule so that the dorsal capsule can be clearly defined. Reconstruction of the scapholunate ligament is recommended along with dorsal capsulodesis using whichever technique is preferred by the surgeon. With the Blatt capsulodesis, the dorsal capsule is elevated using two longitudinal incisions parallel with the axis of the scaphoid.

FIGURE 11

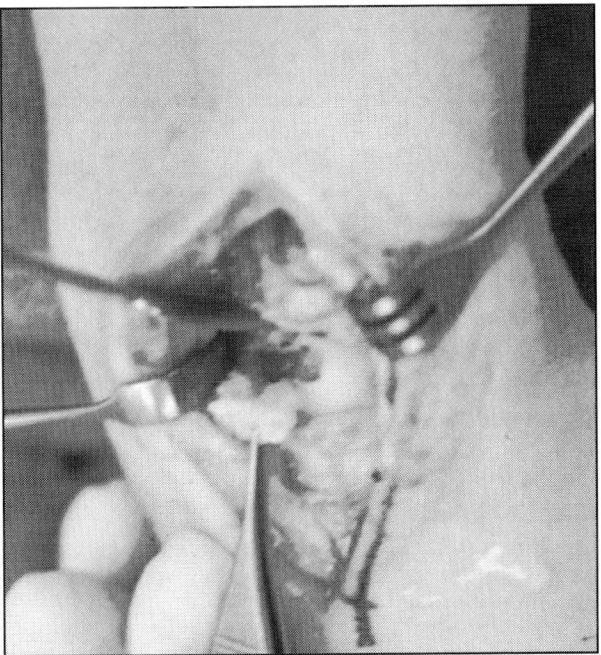

A bone-ligament-bone block is inserted into a site prepared in the dorsum of the scaphoid and lunate. (Reproduced with permission from Trumble TE (ed): *Principles of Hand Surgery and Therapy*. Philadelphia, PA, WB Saunders, 2000, p 110.)

FIGURE 12

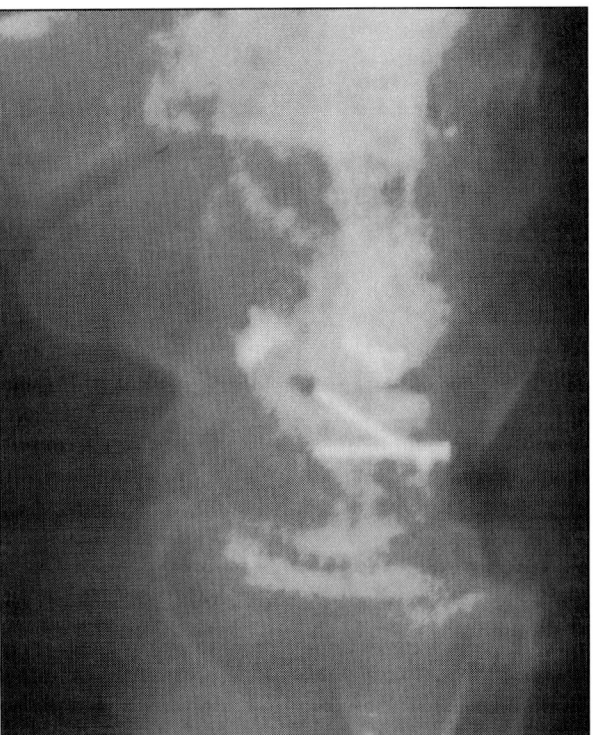

Small screws can be used to secure the bone-ligament-bone graft to the scaphoid and lunate. (Reproduced with permission from Trumble TE (ed): *Principles of Hand Surgery and Therapy*. Philadelphia, PA, WB Saunders, 2000, p 110.)

The strip of capsule is detached from the distal pole of the scaphoid, and a vertical Kirschner wire (K-wire) can be used to assist with correction of scaphoid rotation. The strip of dorsal capsule is then advanced distally and secured to the distal pole of the scaphoid with suture anchors.

Lavernia and associates[11] modified the Blatt procedure to include a repair of the SLIL in addition to the capsulodesis because they found the dorsal capsulodesis alone did not provide sufficient stability of the SLIL. The strip of capsule can be folded back upon itself proximally to expose the ruptured scaphoid interosseous ligament. Their initial procedure called for using drill holes through the scaphoid so that the sutures could be tied over a button on the palmar surface of the wrist, but the development of miniature suture anchors has greatly facilitated this technique.

Berger's Technique Another modification was described by Berger,[1,2] who recommended leaving the capsule attached to the scaphoid distally and then advancing the capsule or attachment on the radius. This allows the capsule to be securely anchored with more exposure than that provided with the distal advancement into the distal pole of the scaphoid (Fig. 9). With this procedure, a flap of dorsal capsule is elevated and left attached to the scaphoid using two parallel incisions in the dorsal intercarpal (DIC) ligament. The dorsal radiocarpal (DRC) ligament is partially divided to expose the ruptured SLIL. Again, K-wires are used as joysticks to align the scaphoid. In placing the suture anchors, it may be more practical to first tie the suture anchors while maintaining the scaphoid alignment with the joysticks before advancing the capsule proximally.

Later Study An additional modification was described in a biomechanical study by Slater and associates.[14] They rotated the DIC ligament in order to attach it along the radial surface of the scaphoid. This modification not only corrects scaphoid rotation but also prevents scaphoid translation radially away from the lunate. In this procedure, the ligament is detached from its point of insertion on the trapezium and distal pole of the scaphoid and ele-

FIGURE 13

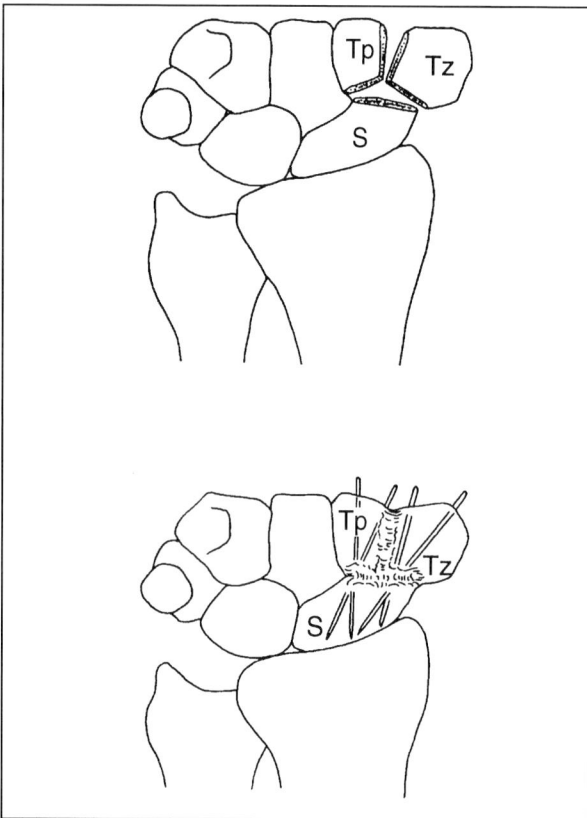

K-wires driven from the trapezoid (Tp) and the trapezium (Tz) stabilize the STT arthrodesis. S = scaphoid. (Reproduced with permission from Trumble TE (ed): *Principles of Hand Surgery and Therapy.* Philadelphia, PA, WB Saunders, 2000, p 112.)

sue through the distal extent of the same incision using the second or third carpometacarpal ligament (Fig. 11). A matching segment of bone is removed from the exposed dorsal surface of the scaphoid and the lunate, and the harvested bone-ligament-bone block is keyed into position and secured with 1.0-mm cortical screws (Fig. 12). Biomechanical studies have demonstrated that these bone-ligament-bone reconstructions can equal or exceed the strength of the native ligament.[16] Although we have had success with these ligament reconstructions for dynamic instability, we have not been able to correct chronic static SLIL injuries with these techniques.

Closure and Postoperative Rehabilitation The fourth dorsal compartment is loosely approximated to the second dorsal compartment, and the skin is closed in layers. Postoperative immobilization requires casting in a long arm spica cast for 1 month and a short arm spica cast for a second month, followed by therapy focusing on active motion for the first month and passive motion in the second month.

Chronic Injuries With Static Instability and Without Arthritic Degeneration

These injuries are among the most challenging wrist ligament injuries to treat surgically. Not only may the primary repair of the SLIL be impossible, but also the scaphoid may be either irreducible or difficult to maintain in the reduced postion required to perform a ligament reconstruction and capsular flap. This is because over time, adjacent uninjured ligaments and wrist capsular tissue shorten, holding the scaphoid flexed and the lunate extended. Wyrick and associates[17] found a high failure rate, with recurrent gapping between the scaphoid and lunate, after ligament reconstruction in this more chronic setting.

Because of the failure of ligament reconstruction to stabilize the wrist, Watson and associates[18] recommended a partial wrist arthrodesis with a fusion of the scaphoid, trapezium, and trapezoid (STT procedure, also referred to as the triscaphe arthrodesis). Others recommend arthrodesis of the scaphoid to the capitate.[19]

STT Procedure The STT procedure can be performed using a longitudinal or a transverse incision at the level just distal to the radial styloid. With a longitudinal incision, the bone graft can be conveniently performed through the same approach as the STT fusion, whereas with the transverse incision, occasionally a separate transverse incision is required to harvest bone graft from the distal radius. Bone graft can be harvested from the iliac crest as

vated using parallel incisions along the DIC ligament (Fig. 10). A portion of the DRC ligament may need to be divided to repair the SLIL with suture anchors. The radial end of the ligament is then advanced and anchored to the proximal radial portion of the scaphoid using suture anchors. Slater and associates showed that biomechanical loading produced less separation between the scaphoid and lunate than does the classic Blatt procedure.

Ligament Grafts If insufficient SLIL remains to allow for primary repair, it may be reconstructed using any of a number of bone-ligament-bone grafts or similar procedures. Weiss[15] demonstrated the use of bone-ligament-bone block harvested from Lister's tubercle to include the retinaculum of the third dorsal compartment. In a modification of the technique described by Weiss, Harvey and associates[16] harvested a bone-ligament-bone block of tis-

FIGURE 14

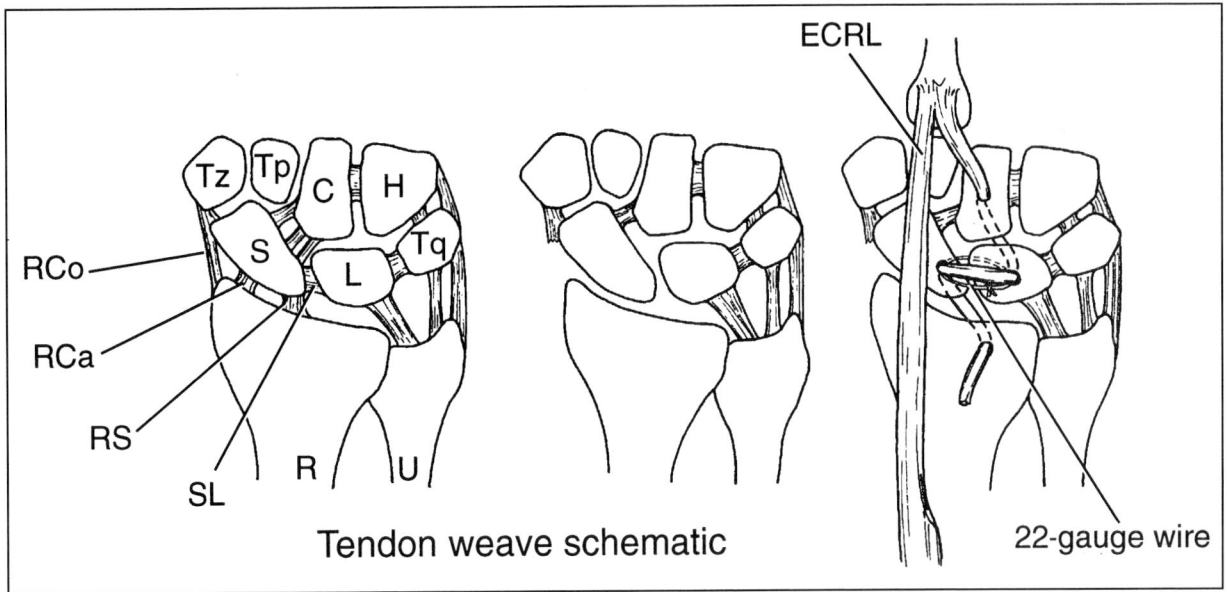

By weaving a strip of the ECRL through the capitate, lunate, scaphoid, and radius, the gapping between the scaphoid and lunate can be corrected. Tz = trapezium, Tp = trapezoid, C = capitate, H = hamate, S = scaphoid, L = lunate, Tq = triquetrum, RCo = radial collateral ligament, RCa = radiocapitate ligament, RS = radioscaphoid ligament, SL = scapholunate interosseous ligament, R = radius, U = ulna. (Reproduced with permission from Trumble TE (ed): *Principles of Hand Surgery and Therapy*. Philadelphia, PA, WB Saunders, 2000, p 111.)

well. The incision is carried down through the skin, and the third dorsal compartment is released so that it can be retracted radially. The STT joint capsule has an overlying fat pad that must be incised with cautery of dorsal blood vessels. The dorsal capsule is incised longitudinally, and flaps are elevated to both the radial and ulnar sides. Curettes and a power burr can be used to decorticate the surfaces of the STT joint. Care is taken to remove all the cartilage down to the palmar recess of the STT joint. Two longitudinal 0.045-inch K-wires are placed in the trapezoid, directed toward the scaphoid, and two pins in the trapezuim are directed toward the scaphoid (Fig. 13). The pins are backed up so they do not obstruct the joint space that has been denuded of cartilage. Bone graft is then harvested from either the distal radius or the iliac crest and packed into the space between the trapezium, trapezoid, and scaphoid to augment the rate of fusion. Once the space has been thoroughly packed with bone graft, the surgeon places pressure on the distal pole of the trapezium to extend the scaphoid and compress it against the trapezoid and trapezium as the wrist is gently deviated radially to further compress the STT joint. The K-wires are then driven into the distal pole of the scaphoid and the alignment confirmed under fluoroscopy. The K-wires can be left protruding from the skin or cut flush and removed at a later point. To avoid impingement between the scaphoid and lunate, a radial styloidectomy is performed. The capsule is repaired loosely with interrupted sutures; the third dorsal compartment is not repaired. The skin is closed in layers.

A long arm spica cast is used for 1 month, followed by a short arm-thumb spica cast for an additional 2 to 3 weeks, until the fusion has incorporated completely. The wires are removed later, either in the surgeon's office or as a minor surgical procedure in the hospital. These arthrodeses limit wrist motion, thereby reducing symptoms of instability and theoretically delaying the progression of arthritic degeneration. However, the STT arthrodesis prevents all normal scaphoid rotation and produces abnormal wrist mechanics, leading to an increased radiocarpal contact pressure.[20]

Tendon Weave Techniques Almquist and associates[21] reported on a tendon weave technique that incorporates the capitate and radius in addition to the lunate and scaphoid to correct static dorsal intercalated segment instability pattern injuries. A follow-up study showed that the tenodesis reduced the scapholunate gap and decreased the progression of traumatic arthritis.

A modification of the procedure by Almquist and associates uses the extensor carpi radialis longus (ECRL) instead of the extensor carpi radialis brevis (ECRB) (Fig. 14). This modified procedure uses a longitudinal dorsal incision that is similar to the exposure for the STT joint except that the entire carpus is exposed through a longitudinal capsular incision. A second longitudinal incision is made along the junction of the radial border of the forearm, between the middle and proximal thirds, in the area where the ECRL can be palpated by placing the distal portion of the tendon under tension. Once the dissection extends down to the interval between the ECRB and the ECRL, the ECRL is carefully identified and partially transected. The strip of the ECRL can then be brought out through the distal incision. Fluoroscopy is used to guide the placement of a cannulated 3.2-mm drill bit in order to accurately place the drill holes through the center of the capitate head, the center of the lunate, the proximal pole of the scaphoid aligned across from the center of the lunate, and through the radius at a point adjacent to the subchondral bone but ulnar to the exit point from the scaphoid. The tension in the tendon graft applies a translational force compressing the scaphoid to the lunate. A folded 22-gauge wire is then used to pass the tendon dorsal to palmar through the capitate, palmar to dorsal through the lunate, dorsal to palmar through the scaphoid, and palmar to dorsal through the radius. An extended carpal tunnel incision is used with the flexor tendons and median nerve gently retracted radially to provide the exposure to retrieve the tendon when it is passed palmar during the tendon weave. It is important to visualize the guide wire and the drill bit as the drill holes are made from dorsal to palmar so that no tendons or nerves are damaged. A cerclage wire is passed from dorsal to palmar through the scaphoid and then back through the lunate from palmar to dorsal, so this can be tensioned by twisting the ends exiting dorsally from the scaphoid and lunate. The tendon graft is placed under tension to take out all the slack before the cerclage wire is tightened. The cerclage wire completely reduces the scaphoid to the lunate. The tendon is then anchored to the radius proximally using either suture anchors or sutures placed with drill holes in the radius. Before completing the ligament repair, we recommend direct repair of any remnants of the SLIL using small suture anchors. The excess portion of the tendon graft is excised. The dorsal capsule is closed, and the dorsal and palmar skin incisions are closed in layers.

A long arm-thumb spica cast is used for 6 weeks, followed by a short arm spica cast for an additional month.

Although the cerclage wire frequently breaks as the patient regains wrist motion, the wire usually does not need to be removed. According to Almquist and associates,[21] the tendon graft will maintain most of the correction of the scapholunate interval space, although some widening will occur from the initial postoperative reduction.

Brunelli and Brunelli[22] have described stabilization of the rotated scaphoid with a slip of the flexor carpi radialis, but we have no experience with the procedure. One comparison of STT arthrodesis and the four-bone weave showed that the weave technique resulted in more nearly normal radiocarpal contact characteristics.[23] However, few other outcomes studies are available to assist the surgeon in choosing between a weave technique and an intercarpal fusion when treating a chronic static scapholunate dissociation without arthritic changes. Our preference is to use the STT fusion for patients older than 40 years of age and the Almquist procedure for patients younger than 40 years of age. This is an arbitrary determination, and all the procedures require a thorough discussion of risks and benefits with the patient.

Chronic Instability With Degenerative Changes and Fixed Rotation of the Scaphoid

Finally, for patients with chronic scapholunate instability associated with degenerative changes and fixed rotation of the scaphoid, soft-tissue reconstruction is no longer an option. Limited arthrodeses that incorporate the scaphoid are also contraindicated because they fail to address the radiocarpal arthritis. The most commonly recommended treatment options in this late setting are excision of the scaphoid with associated intercarpal arthrodesis of the capitate, hamate, lunate, and triquetrum (the so-called "four-corner fusion" or SLAC wrist procedure)[24] and proximal row carpectomy. These procedures yield roughly equivalent results in terms of pain relief and decreased range of motion. Total wrist fusion is usually held in reserve, to be used in the event of failure of one of the procedures described earlier.[25,26]

CONCLUSION

The availability of so many distinct procedures and the continual development of new techniques suggest that no single treatment algorithm is optimal for the entire spectrum of SLIL injuries. Surgeon preference probably plays as great a role as any factor. Outcomes research in this area is ongoing and will be useful to all who treat these challenging injuries.

REFERENCES

1. Berger RA: The gross and histologic anatomy of the scapholunate interosseous ligament. *J Hand Surg Am* 1996;21:170-178.

2. Berger RA, Imeada T, Berglund L, An KN: Constraint and material properties of the subregions of the scapholunate interosseous ligament. *J Hand Surg Am* 1999;24:953-962.

3. Watson HK, Ballet FL: The SLAC wrist: Scapholunate advanced collapse pattern of degenerative arthritis. *J Hand Surg Am* 1984;9:358-365.

4. Mayfield JK, Johnson RP, Kilcoyne RF: The ligaments of the human wrist and their functional significance. *Anat Rec* 1976;186:417-428.

5. Watson HK, Ashmead D IV, Makhlouf MV: Examination of the scaphoid. *J Hand Surg Am* 1988;13:657-660.

6. Linscheid RL, Dobyns JH, Beabout JW, Bryan RS: Traumatic instability of the wrist: Diagnosis, classification, and pathomechanics. *J Bone Joint Surg Am* 1972;54:1612-1632.

7. Belsole RJ, Quinn SF, Greene TL, Beatty ME, Rayhack JM: Digital subtraction arthrography of the wrist. *J Bone Joint Surg Am* 1990;72:846-851.

8. Pin PG, Semenkovich JW, Young VL, et al: Role of radionuclide imaging in the evaluation of wrist pain. *J Hand Surg Am* 1988;13:810-814.

9. Johnstone DJ, Thorogood S, Smith WH, Scott TD: A comparison of magnetic resonance imaging and arthroscopy in the investigation of chronic wrist pain. *J Hand Surg Br* 1997;22:714-718.

10. Geissler WB, Freeland AE, Savoie FH, McIntyre LW, Whipple TL: Intracarpal soft-tissue lesions associated with an intra-articular fracture of the distal end of the radius. *J Bone Joint Surg Am* 1996;78:357-365.

11. Lavernia CJ, Cohen MS, Taleisnik J: Treatment of scapholunate dissociation by ligamentous repair and capsulodesis. *J Hand Surg Am* 1992;17:354-359.

12. Trumble TE (ed): *Principles of Hand Surgery and Therapy.* Philadelphia, PA, WB Saunders, 2000, p 106.

13. Blatt G: Capsulodesis in reconstructive hand surgery: Dorsal capsulodesis for the unstable scaphoid and volar capsulodesis following excision of the distal ulna. *Hand Clin* 1987;3:81-102.

14. Slater RR Jr, Szabo RM, Bay BK, Laubach J: Dorsal intercarpal ligament capsulodesis for scapholunate dissociation: Biomechanical analysis in a cadaver model. *J Hand Surg Am* 1999;24:232-239.

15. Weiss AP: Scapholunate ligament reconstruction using a bone-retinaculum-bone autograft. *J Hand Surg Am* 1998;23:205-215.

16. Harvey EJ, Hanel D, Knight JB, Tencer AF: Autograft replacements for the scapholunate ligament: A biomechanical comparison of hand-based autografts. *J Hand Surg Am* 1999;24:963-967.

17. Wyrick JD, Youse BD, Kiefhaber TR: Scapholunate ligament repair and capsulodesis for the treatment of static scapholunate dissociation. *J Hand Surg Br* 1998;23:776-780.

18. Watson HK, Ryu J, Akelman E: Limited triscaphoid intercarpal arthrodesis for rotatory subluxation of the scaphoid. *J Bone Joint Surg Am* 1986;68:345-349.

19. Pisano SM, Peimer CA, Wheeler DR, Sherwin F: Scaphocapitate intercarpal arthrodesis. *J Hand Surg Am* 1991;16:328-333.

20. Viegas SF, Patterson RM, Peterson PD, et al: Evaluation of the biomechanical efficacy of limited intercarpal fusions for the treatment of scapholunate dissociation. *J Hand Surg Am* 1990;15:120-128.

21. Almquist EE, Bach AW, Sack JT, Fuhs SE, Newman DM: Four-bone ligament reconstruction for treatment of chronic complete scapholunate separation. *J Hand Surg Am* 1991;16:322-327.

22. Brunelli GA, Brunelli GR: A new technique to correct carpal instability with scaphoid rotary subluxation: A preliminary report. *J Hand Surg Am* 1995;20:S82-S85.

23. Augsburger S, Necking L, Horton J, Bach AW, Tencer AF: A comparison of scaphoid-trapezium-trapezoid fusion and four-bone tendon weave for scapholunate dissociation. *J Hand Surg Am* 1992;17:360-369.

24. Ashmead D IV, Watson HK, Damon C, Herber S, Paly W: Scapholunate advanced collapse wrist salvage. *J Hand Surg Am* 1994;19:741-750.

25. Wyrick JD, Stern PJ, Kiefhaber TR: Motion-preserving procedures in the treatment of scapholunate advanced collapse wrist: Proximal row carpectomy versus four-corner arthrodesis. *J Hand Surg Am* 1995;20:965-970.

26. Cohen MS, Kozin SH: Degenerative arthritis of the wrist: Proximal row carpectomy versus scaphoid excision and four-corner arthrodesis. *J Hand Surg Am* 2001;26:94-104.

CHAPTER 6

TRANSSCAPHOID PERILUNATE DISLOCATIONS

THOMAS E. TRUMBLE, MD

Lunate, perilunate, and transscaphoid perilunate fracture-dislocations represent a spectrum of injuries that are defined according to where the line of injury travels through the wrist (Fig. 1). These injuries usually occur in young people and typically involve high-energy trauma. In the perilunate dislocation, the line of injury first travels through the scapholunate interosseous ligament (SLIL) and then through the capsular ligaments surrounding the lunocapitate articulation (involving the radioscaphocapitate and ulnocapitate ligaments), completing the injury through the carpus by disrupting the lunotriquetral interosseous ligament (LTIL).[1,2]

FIGURE 1

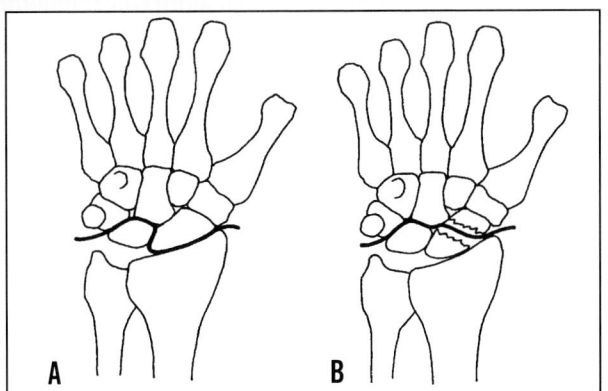

Lines of injury in lunate, perilunate, and transscaphoid perilunate fracture-dislocations. **A,** With perilunate and lunate dislocations, the line of injury causes disruption of the scapholunate interosseous ligament (SLIL) and the lunotriquetral interosseous ligament (LTIL). **B,** In transscaphoid perilunate fracture-dislocations, the injury causes a fracture of the scaphoid instead of disrupting the SLIL. These injuries also include a disruption of the LTIL. (Reproduced with permission from Trumble TE (ed): *Principles of Hand Surgery and Therapy.* Philadelphia, PA, WB Saunders, 2000, p 112.)

In transscaphoid perilunate fracture-dislocations, the line of injury travels through the scaphoid, resulting in a fracture (Fig. 2). In most cases, the proximal pole of the scaphoid remains attached to the lunate because the SLIL remains intact. The results of treatment for transscaphoid fracture-dislocations are generally better than for perilunate dislocations because the fracture can heal to restore normal wrist kinematics, whereas in perilunate injuries the SLIL repair never results in normal function.

ASSOCIATED INJURIES AND TREATMENT PRINCIPLES

Because most transscaphoid perilunate dislocations occur in high-energy scenarios, the physician must remember to follow basic life support measures first. Furthermore, it is important to conduct a complete musculoskeletal examination, including a careful spine evaluation, rather than focusing exclusively on any obvious, significant wrist deformity.

Median nerve injuries can occur by a direct blow, such as a contusion, or secondarily, from bleeding and increased pressure within the carpal tunnel. Patients with an immediate median nerve deficit following an injury probably do not need nerve decompression acutely because the decompression will not correct the deficit. However, if the neurologic deficit progresses or if median nerve symptoms develop late (suggesting increasing pressure in the carpal canal), decompression of the carpal tunnel should be done on an urgent basis.

Concomitant distal radius fractures also may occur, particularly radial styloid fractures and dorsal rim fractures, because the line of injury produces a shear fracture of the radius rather than a disruption of the radiocarpal liga-

FIGURE 2

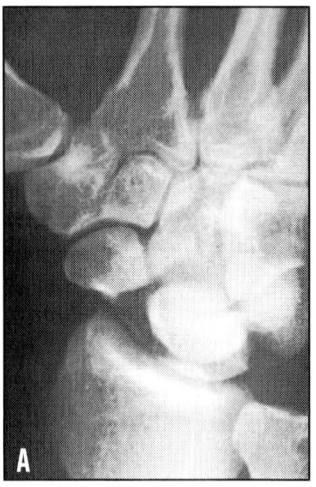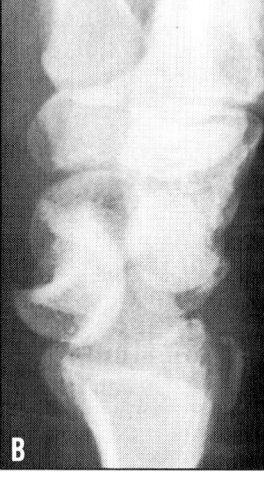

Radiographs of a transscaphoid perilunate fracture-dislocation. **A,** This oblique radiograph helps to identify the injury to the scaphoid. The proximal pole of the scaphoid has displaced with the lunate. **B,** This lateral radiograph shows the capitate displaced dorsal to the lunate with the lunate still in the lunate fossa of the distal radius. (Reproduced with permission from Trumble TE (ed): *Principles of Hand Surgery and Therapy.* Philadelphia, PA, WB Saunders, 2000, p 115.)

FIGURE 3

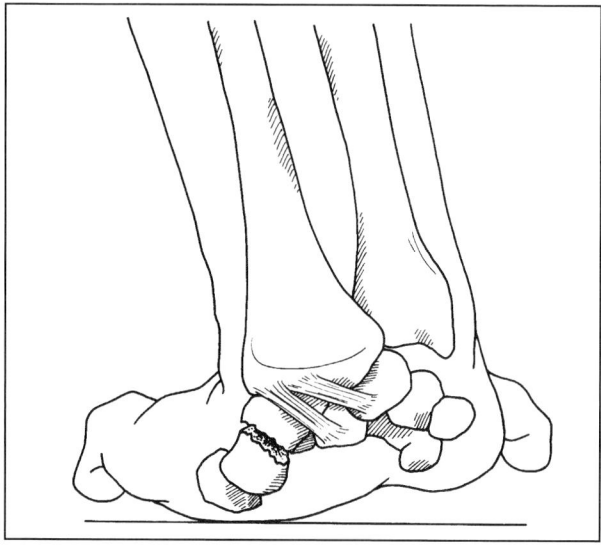

Mechanism of injury in scaphoid fracture. The angle of wrist extension and radial deviation determines whether the scaphoid fractures or the SLIL is disrupted. (Reproduced with permission from Trumble TE (ed): *Principles of Hand Surgery and Therapy.* Philadelphia, PA, WB Saunders, 2000, p 93.)

ments. These injuries should be anatomically reduced and stabilized with internal fixation when addressing the perilunate component of the injury.

BIOMECHANICAL ROLE OF THE SCAPHOID

The scaphoid is the key to the carpus because it allows both tremendous mobility of the wrist in flexion/extension and radial/ulnar deviation and provides stability as the intercalated segment linking the proximal and the distal carpal rows. Much of the wrist motion is a result of rotation of the scaphoid and the rest of the proximal row during radial and ulnar deviation. The scaphoid rotates to become more vertical, or colinear with the radius, with ulnar deviation bringing the lunate and triquetrum into dorsal rotation (ie, the distal surface of the bone rotates dorsally). The scaphoid can be thought of as working like a crank handle to drive the rotation of the lunate and triquetrum. With radial deviation, the scaphoid rotates to become more horizontal, or perpendicular to the long axis of the radius. The dorsal intercalated segmental instability (DISI) pattern occurs with disruption of the SLIL, causing the distal surface of the lunate to tilt dorsally. The volar intercalated segment instability (VISI) injury pat-

tern occurs with disruption of the LTIL, the capitolunate ligament (volar arcuate), and the dorsal radiotriquetral ligament.[3-5] With this complex linkage in the wrist, it is not surprising that the center of rotation for flexion/extension is different from that of radial/ulnar deviation. For both planes of motion, the center moves slightly as the wrist moves, describing a centroid pattern.

RADIOGRAPHIC PARAMETERS

The carpus maintains a constant ratio between the height of the third metacarpal and the carpus (0.54 ± 0.03)[6] (see Fig. 9 in chapter 4). A decrease in the ratio indicates a collapse of the scaphoid or instability of the ligaments of the proximal row (eg, the SLIL is disrupted and allows proximal migration of the capitate). The carpal bones also maintain a fairly constant angle of alignment with respect to one another. The normal scapholunate angle averages 46° (range, 30° to 60°). The capitolunate and the radiolunate angles each average 0° (range, −15° to 15°). With a disruption of the SLIL or with a palmar collapse of the scaphoid because of a fracture, the scapholunate angle increases as the distal surface of the lunate rotates dorsally with respect to the scaphoid. These parameters are important for reviewing plain radiographs; however, tri-

FIGURE 4

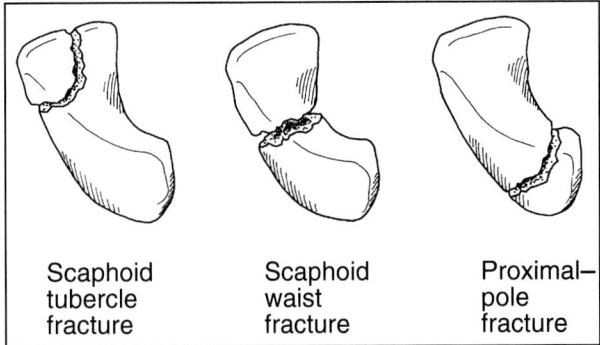

Scaphoid fractures can be classified as scaphoid tubercle fractures, scaphoid waist fractures, and proximal-pole fractures. (Reproduced with permission from Trumble TE (ed): *Principles of Hand Surgery and Therapy*. Philadelphia, PA, WB Saunders, 2000, p 93.)

FIGURE 5

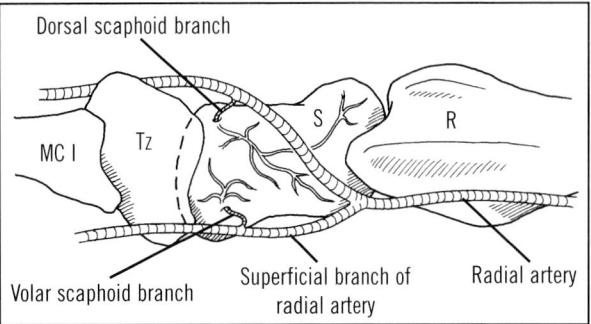

Blood supply to the scaphoid is based primarily on dorsal branches of the radial artery that perforate the radial and dorsal cortex of the scaphoid near the waist of the scaphoid. (Reproduced with permission from Trumble TE (ed): *Principles of Hand Surgery and Therapy*. Philadelphia, PA, WB Saunders, 2000, p 94.)

spiral CT is the most reliable method of assessing transscaphoid injuries in terms of evaluating fracture patterns and comminution.

SCAPHOID FRACTURES ASSOCIATED WITH TRANSSCAPHOID PERILUNATE FRACTURE-DISLOCATIONS

When the hand is outstretched and the wrist is in ulnar deviation, the scaphoid is vertically aligned. The axial load combined with the normal palmar curvature of the scaphoid results in a bending moment that collapses the scaphoid (Fig. 3). The fracture can involve the scaphoid waist, proximal pole, or the tubercle; waist fractures are the type most commonly associated with transscaphoid perilunate fracture-dislocations (Fig. 4). Proximal-pole fractures have the poorest prognosis because blood supply to the proximal pole is disrupted by the fracture. In these injuries it is important to identify whether or not the fracture is comminuted because such fractures may require bone grafting with internal fixation, requiring a different surgical approach. As mentioned, trispiral CT is currently the most reliable means of assessing fracture configuration and the amount of comminution.

Understanding scaphoid anatomy is essential for treating transscaphoid perilunate injuries. *Scaphoid* is Greek for "canoe" or "boat"; the scaphoid actually resembles a bent and twisted boat. The plane of the scaphoid, which is 45° of palmar tilt to the longitudinal axis of the forearm and 45° radial angulation from the central axis of the forearm

on the PA projection, often deceives surgeons. The entire proximal half of the scaphoid is an articular surface within the radiocarpal joint, so the blood supply can enter only on the distal palmar segments and dorsal ridge. Vessels entering the dorsal ridge of the scaphoid arise directly from the radial artery and supply 70% to 80% of the bone, including the proximal pole (Fig. 5). For this reason, proximal-pole fractures require the longest time to union (as long as 10 months) and are associated with a high incidence of osteonecrosis (approaching 50%). Approximately one third of patients have no perforating vessels proximal to the scaphoid waist.

TREATMENT

For patients with perilunate or equivalent injuries, open reduction and internal fixation with acute ligament repair is recommended because late carpal instability invariably occurs with closed treatment.[7] However, closed reduction should be performed urgently to optimize the carpal alignment and reduce the pressure on the median nerve until the patient can undergo surgery. Nearly all of these dislocations occur with the capitate displaced dorsally. The carpus should be reduced as soon as possible by extending the wrist to recreate the deformity and applying dorsal pressure to reduce the capitate into the lunate fossa (Fig. 6). If the scaphoid has minimal comminution, this injury can be treated with a palmar Russe approach for screw fixation of the scaphoid and percutaneous pin fixation of the lunotriquetral joint.[8] Although several authors recommend Kirschner wire (K-wire) fixation of the scaphoid fracture, screw fixation provides a stable

FIGURE 6

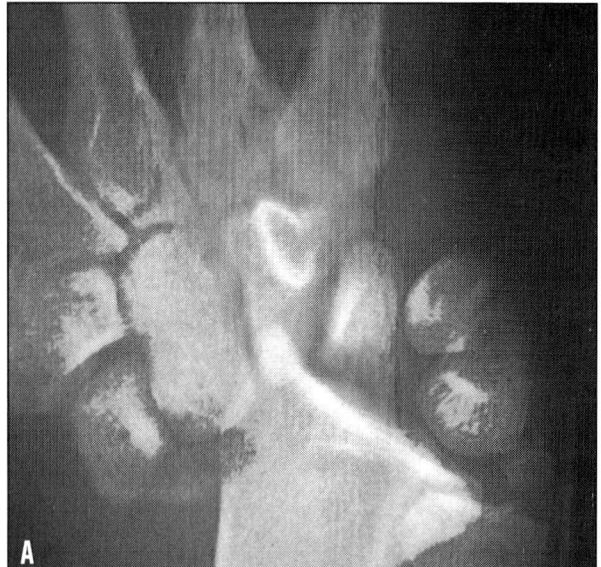

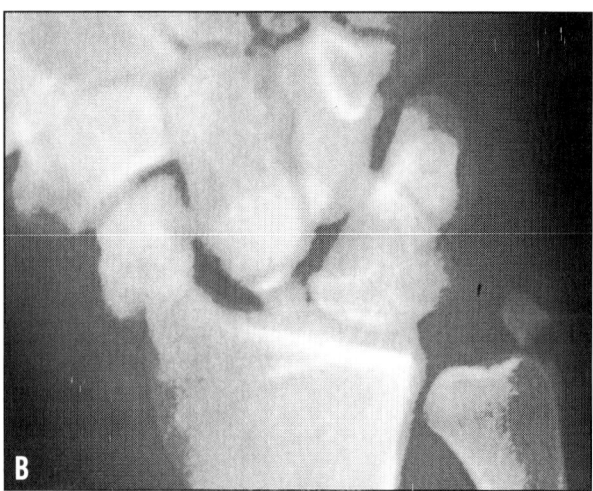

Radiographs showing an extremely displaced transscaphoid perilunate dislocation. **A,** Initial radiograph. **B,** Following closed reduction, the proximal pole is still displaced, along with the lunate, toward the palmar surface. (Reproduced with permission from Trumble TE (ed): *Principles of Hand Surgery and Therapy*. Philadelphia, PA, WB Saunders, 2000, p 116.)

FIGURE 7

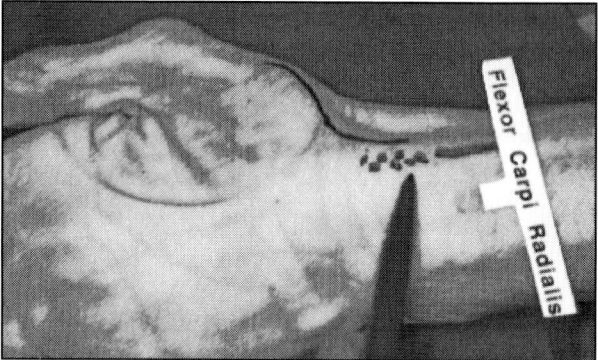

The palmar Russe approach for stabilization of the scaphoid. (Reproduced with permission from Trumble TE (ed): *Principles of Hand Surgery and Therapy*. Philadelphia, PA, WB Saunders, 2000, p 98.)

FIGURE 8

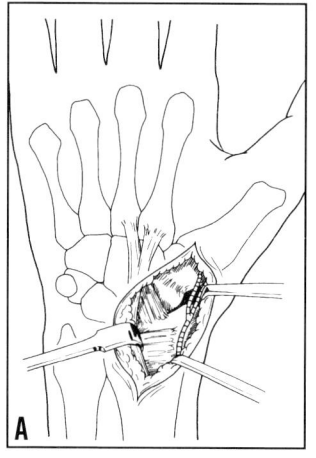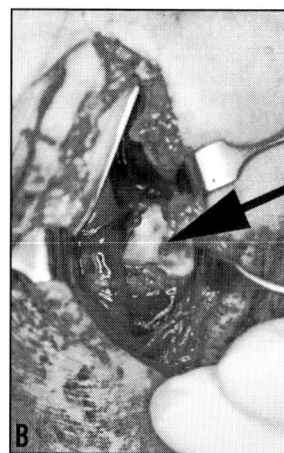

The palmar approach for scaphoid fractures. **A,** The scaphoid fracture is exposed by incising the sheath of the flexor carpi radialis and retracting it ulnarly. The capsule overlying the scaphoid waist and distal polar is incised. Care is taken to try to preserve the RSC ligament. **B,** Photograph of the palmar approach with the displaced proximal pole of the scaphoid seen in the wound (arrow). (Reproduced with permission from Trumble TE (ed): *Principles of Hand Surgery and Therapy*. Philadelphia, PA, WB Saunders, 2000, p 98, p 115.)

construct with a permanent implant that allows early motion. A dorsal approach with retrograde screw fixation of the scaphoid is recommended (1) when the scaphoid remains significantly displaced despite an initial closed reduction, (2) when the lunotriquetral articulation is unstable to stress under fluoroscopy, or (3) when the comminution of the scaphoid involves a significant portion of the scaphoid waist; this is because the dorsal approach provides the necessary exposure to realign the scaphoid (often with bone grafting) and repair the LTIL.

Palmar Approach

Incision and Reduction A standard Russe incision is made along the course of the flexor carpi radialis (FCR) and

FIGURE 9

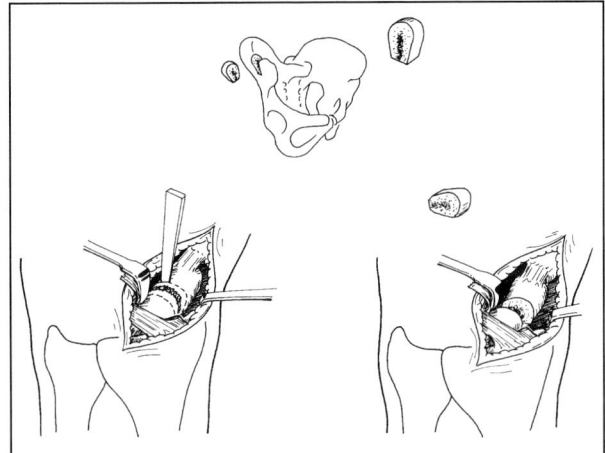

For comminuted fractures with collapse, a bone graft can be added to the palmar approach using bone from the iliac crest or distal radius. (Reproduced with permission from Trumble TE (ed): *Principles of Hand Surgery and Therapy*. Philadelphia, PA, WB Saunders, 2000, p 100.)

FIGURE 10

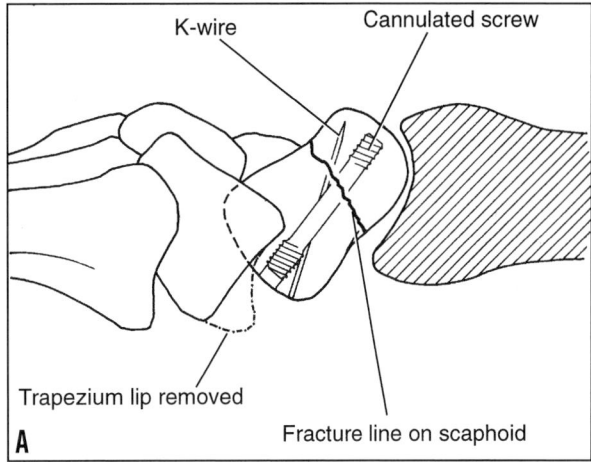

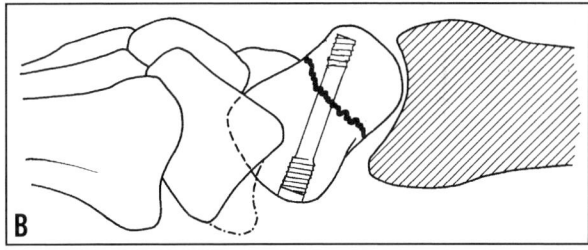

Internal fixation of the scaphoid using the palmar approach as described by Russe. **A,** The palmar lip of the trapezium must be removed to insert the scaphoid screw into the longitudinal axis of the scaphoid. For unstable scaphoid fractures, a K-wire is used prior to screw placement to control rotation. **B,** Failure to remove the palmar rim often results in dorsal placement of the scaphoid screw close to the fracture line, producing a marginal stability. (Reproduced with permission from Trumble TE (ed): *Principles of Hand Surgery and Therapy*. Philadelphia, PA, WB Saunders, 2000, p 101.)

FIGURE 11

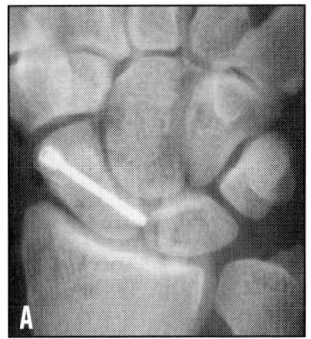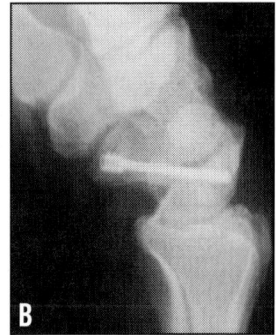

Postoperative radiographs of the transscaphoid perilunate fracture shown in Fig. 2. Stabilization of the scaphoid fracture has been achieved using a Herbert screw. **A,** AP radiograph. **B,** Lateral radiograph. (Reproduced with permission from Trumble TE (ed): *Principles of Hand Surgery and Therapy*. Philadelphia, PA, WB Saunders, 2000, p 115.)

extended distally along the border of the glabrous skin of the thenar eminence (Fig. 7). Splitting the sheath of the FCR allows it to be retracted ulnarly to protect the palmar cutaneous branch of the median nerve. The floor of the FCR sheath is incised longitudinally to the scaphoid (Fig. 8). I try to preserve as much of the radioscaphocapitate (RSC) ligament as possible because this helps to contain the proximal pole and prevent it from subluxating palmarly. Dental picks are favored over K-wire joysticks to avoid propagation of comminution in the fracture fragments. Tricortical bone grafts are used to wedge open collapsed scaphoid fractures to correct their alignment. These grafts may be taken from the iliac crest or the distal radius (Fig. 9). The inner wall of the dorsal scaphoid cortex can be notched with a small osteotome to accommodate the wedge graft. The surgeon must take care not to disrupt the dorsal cortex of the scaphoid, which can detach the blood supply and make the fracture highly unstable. Furthermore, the dorsal cortex continuity serves as a hinge around which the distal fragment can be rotated while it is reduced by a dorsiflexion maneuver. However, I generally prefer the dorsal approach when there is significant comminution.

Screw Fixation of the Scaphoid It is important to remove the small palmar beak of the trapezium with a rongeur to provide the best access for screw insertion into the long axis of the scaphoid. Failure to do so can result in placing the screw at an angle that puts the end of the

FIGURE 12

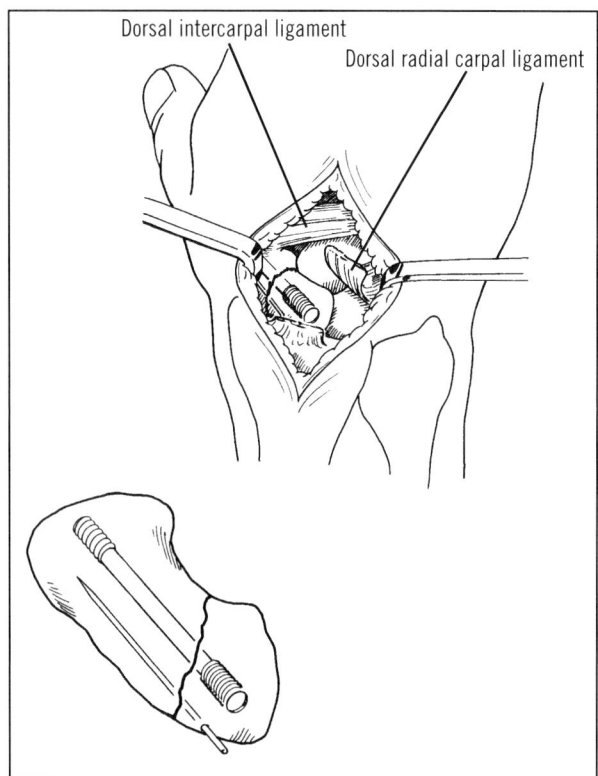

Dorsal approach for stabilizing the scaphoid fracture in a transscaphoid perilunate dislocation. This exposure is extended ulnarly by reflecting the extensor digitorium communis from the dorsal capsule to expose the lunotriquetral articulations so that the LTIL can be repaired. (Reproduced with permission from Trumble TE (ed): *Principles of Hand Surgery and Therapy*. Philadelphia, PA, WB Saunders, 2000, p 101.)

FIGURE 13

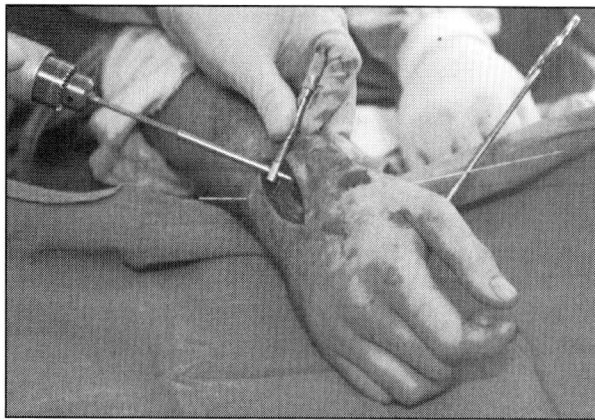

Use of the cannulated system for insertion of the noncannulated Herbert screw. This system greatly improves the accuracy of reduction, particularly when comminution is present. (Reproduced with permission from Trumble TE (ed): *Principles of Hand Surgery and Therapy*. Philadelphia, PA, WB Saunders, 2000, p 116.)

screw too dorsal and near the fracture line[9] (Fig. 10). To measure the length of the screw, the guide is inserted up to the limits of the subchondral bone of the proximal pole. The guide wire is then driven into the radius to prevent it from dislodging, and a cannulated drill and tap are used to prepare the path for the screw while checking views under fluoroscopy. The guide wire helps the surgeon place the screw in the center of the proximal pole, where it will provide the most stable fixation. Once the screw is inserted, the guide wire is removed and plain radiographs are taken to confirm the position of the screw. The palmar capsule is repaired with interrupted sutures, especially if any portion of the RSC ligament has been incised. The subcutaneous layer and skin are closed in separate layers and a long arm plaster splint is applied postoperatively. Two weeks after surgery, the splint and sutures are removed and a short arm cast is applied for 1 month, at which time the cast is discontinued and a removable splint is used until the radiographs confirm union (Fig. 11).

Dorsal Approach

Although the palmar approach is favored for waist fractures because it protects the major vascular supply to the scaphoid, it does not provide adequate exposure to reduce comminuted scaphoid fractures and to repair the LTIL. The dorsal approach can be performed safely as long as the blood supply entering with the cuff of tissue on the dorsal surface of the scaphoid just distal to the articular surface contacting the radius is preserved. In addition to providing better exposure for bone grafting, the dorsal approach also allows for more accurate placement of implants in small proximal-pole fractures.

Incision and Reduction The third dorsal compartment, which contains the extensor pollicis longus, is released, and the extensor pollicis longus is retracted radially (Fig. 12). The extensor carpi radialis longus is retracted radially, and the capsule of the wrist is incised longitudinally to expose the scaphoid. My preference when using the dorsal approach with small proximal-pole fractures has been to insert a noncannulated Herbert screw when possible, because it leaves the smallest footprint in the articular cartilage. However, I use the guide pin and drill for the cannulated screw set to prepare a path for the noncannulated scaphoid screw (Fig. 13). Once the cannulated

FIGURE 14

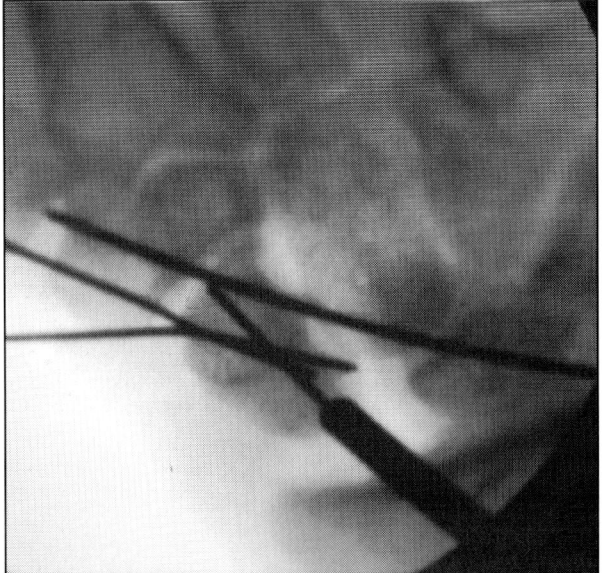

AP fluoroscopy image demonstrates the use of supplemental K-wires to provide the initial stabilization of the scaphoid so that a central guide pin can be placed, overdrilled, and then removed for noncannulated screw fixation.

FIGURE 15

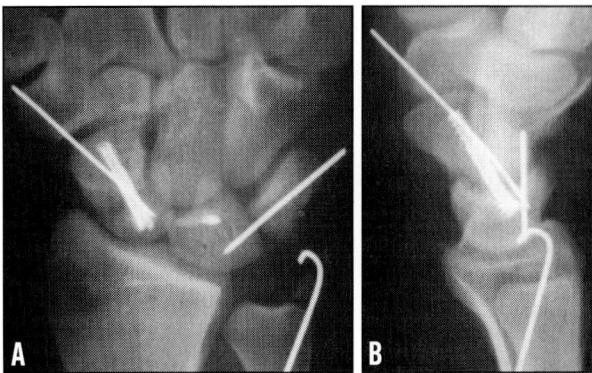

Radiographs demonstrating the postoperative reduction of the transscaphoid perilunate fracture-dislocation shown in Fig. 6. In addition to retrograde screw placement, a supplemental K-wire has been used for stabilization of the scaphoid. The lunotriquetral ligament has been repaired using a suture anchor and a percutaneously placed K-wire. **A,** AP radiograph. **B,** Lateral radiograph demonstrating that the scapholunate angle has been restored with correction of the scaphoid anatomy and restoration of the carpal height. (Reproduced with permission from Trumble TE (ed): *Principles of Hand Surgery and Therapy.* Philadelphia, PA, WB Saunders, 2000, pp 116, 117.)

guide pin has been used to drill and tap the hole, a secondary K-wire is placed parallel to the guide pin to maintain the reduction and to control rotation of the fracture fragments while the guide pin is removed and the Herbert screw is inserted (Fig. 14). When the scaphoid fracture is very unstable, a commuted scaphoid screw can be used. Implants must be countersunk adequately because insertion is performed in the center of the articular surface of the proximal pole.

Ligament Repair After the scaphoid is stabilized, the SLIL is inspected to make sure that it is competent. The SLIL requires repair only rarely, while the LTIL routinely requires repair. The lunotriquetral joint can be exposed by elevating the fourth dorsal compartment off the capsule using sharp dissection. In most cases, the LTIL is avulsed from the lunate. One or two 1.8-mm anchors are inserted into the lunate, and the double-armed sutures are passed through the ligament remaining with the triquetrum. Before tying the sutures, the lunotriquetral articulation is reduced and pinned with a K wire driven percutaneously through the ulnar border of the hand (Fig. 15). In contrast to isolated SLIL injuries and perilunate dislocations, the screw fixation of the scaphoid and the pinning of the LTIL allow for early motion. When the

scaphoid fracture is not comminuted, I recommend splinting the wrist for 2 weeks, until the swelling subsides, before starting early active range-of-motion exercises. Passive exercises are started 6 weeks after surgery. For transscaphoid perilunate injuries with comminuted fractures, the wrist is immobilized for 6 weeks in a short armthumb spica cast. Active exercises are started once the cast has been removed, followed by passive exercises 1 month later.

COMPLICATIONS
Osteonecrosis of the Scaphoid

Some transient loss of vascularity occurs in the proximal pole of most scaphoid fractures associated with carpal dislocation, but early screw fixation helps to facilitate bone ingrowth from the distal pole into the proximal pole of the scaphoid to revascularize the proximal pole. Poor reduction, delayed surgery, and inadequate fixation of the scaphoid can increase the incidence of osteonecrosis and decrease the rate of fracture healing. Recent studies have established the value of MRI in assessing proximal-pole vascularity, although the implants can make it difficult to interpret the MRI postoperatively.[10-13] Revision surgery with vascularized bone grafts may be necessary to promote fracture healing.[14]

FIGURE 16

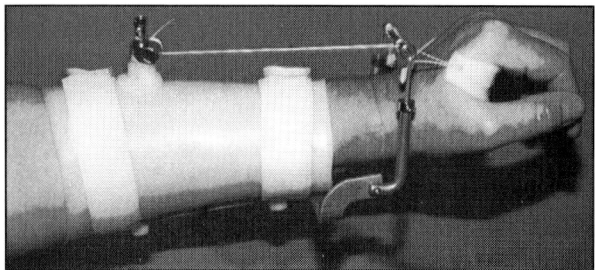

For patients who have persistent wrist stiffness despite a hand therapy program, this static progressive splint helps to increase wrist extension. A similar splint can be made to enhance wrist flexion. (Reproduced with permission from Trumble TE (ed): *Principles of Hand Surgery and Therapy.* Philadelphia, PA, WB Saunders, 2000, p 117.)

Delayed Union and Nonunion of the Scaphoid Fracture

Green[15] demonstrated the association between decreased bone vascularity and decreased healing of scaphoid nonunions. The same factors that help to minimize the risk of severe osteonecrosis also help to promote fracture union. The use of accurately placed screws to compress the fracture site can optimize healing by decreasing motion and gapping at the fracture site. Most nonunions that develop despite adequate fixation are associated with osteonecrosis and should be treated by a vascularized bone graft as described earlier if the articular surfaces are preserved.

Late VISI of the Carpus

The LTIL, in addition to the dorsal radioscaphotriquetral ligament, plays an important role in VISI injuries.[5] The best way to prevent VISI deformity is to adequately repair the LTIL. Late cases of VISI deformities can be treated with a dorsal capsulodesis involving the lunate and triquetrum or an ulnar four-bone arthrodesis.[5,16]

Wrist Stiffness

Nearly all patients with transscaphoid perilunate fracture-dislocations will experience some decrease in wrist motion. Stable fixation in these injuries allows for early range-of-motion exercises, which may reduce the loss of motion. Static progressive splints can help certain patients regain motion postoperatively (Fig. 16).

Wrist Arthrosis

There are no long-term studies of transscaphoid perilunate fracture-dislocations. In a number of cases, articular damage to the scaphoid or radius has been shown to be the inciting event for wrist degeneration. Osteonecrosis, poor reduction, and inadequate stabilization of the scaphoid can result in wrist arthrosis. In these cases, salvage procedures such as proximal row carpectomy or partial wrist arthrodesis can relieve pain and still allow some motion. In severe cases, a total wrist arthrodesis may be required.

REFERENCES

1. Mayfield JK: Mechanism of carpal injuries. *Clin Orthop* 1980;149:45-54.
2. Mayfield JK, Johnson RP, Kilcoyne RK: Carpal dislocations: Pathomechanics and progressive perilunar instability. *J Hand Surg Am* 1980;5:226-241.
3. Linscheid RL, Dobyns JH: The unified concept of carpal injuries. *Ann Chir Main* 1984;3:35-42.
4. Linscheid RL, Dobyns JH, Beckenbaugh RD, Cooney WP III, Wood MB: Instability patterns of the wrist. *J Hand Surg Am* 1983;8:682-686.
5. Trumble TE, Bour CJ, Smith RJ, Glisson RR: Kinematics of the ulnar carpus related to the volar intercalated segment instability pattern. *J Hand Surg Am* 1990;15:384-392.
6. Youm Y, Yoon YS: Analytical development in investigation of wrist kinematics. *J Biomech* 1979;12:613-621.
7. Minami A, Kaneda K: Repair and/or reconstruction of scapholunate interosseous ligament in lunate and perilunate dislocations. *J Hand Surg Am* 1993;18:1099-1106.
8. Viegas SF, Bean JW, Schram RA: Transscaphoid fracture/dislocations treated with open reduction and Herbert screw internal fixation. *J Hand Surg Am* 1987;12:992-999.
9. Trumble TE, Clarke T, Kreder HJ: Non-union of the scaphoid: Treatment with cannulated screws compared with treatment with Herbert screws. *J Bone Joint Surg Am* 1996;78:1829-1837.
10. Morgan WJ, Breen TF, Coumas JM, Schulz LA: Role of magnetic resonance imaging in assessing factors affecting healing in scaphoid nonunions. *Clin Orthop* 1997;336:240-246.
11. Perlik PC, Guilford WB: Magnetic resonance imaging to assess vascularity of scaphoid nonunions. *J Hand Surg Am* 1991;16:479-484.
12. Sakuma M, Nakamura R, Imaeda T: Analysis of proximal fragment sclerosis and surgical outcome of scaphoid nonunion by magnetic resonance imaging. *J Hand Surg Br* 1995;20:201-205.
13. Trumble TE: Avascular necrosis after scaphoid fracture: A correlation of magnetic resonance imaging and histology. *J Hand Surg Am* 1990;15:557-564.

14. Zaidemberg C, Siebert JW, Angrigiani C: A new vascular-ized bone graft for scaphoid nonunion. *J Hand Surg Am* 1991;16:474-47816.

15. Green DP: The effect of avascular necrosis on Russe bone grafting for scaphoid nonunion. *J Hand Surg Am* 1985; 10:597-605.

16. Trumble TE, Bour CJ, Smith RJ, Edwards GS: Intercarpal arthrodesis for static and dynamic volar intercalated segment instability. *J Hand Surg Am* 1988;3:384-390.

CHAPTER 7

CAPITATE AND TRIQUETRUM FRACTURE-DISLOCATIONS

ERIC P. HOFMEISTER, MD
ALEXANDER Y. SHIN, MD

The human wrist is a highly mobile joint that augments the mechanical strength of the digits while transmitting the torque generated by the forearm. The anatomy that makes this great mobility possible also makes it highly susceptible to injuries, especially loading injuries to a dorsiflexed wrist. Of the perilunate injuries associated with fractures, the most common fracture patterns are the transradius and transscaphoid variants. The transcapitate, transtriquetral, and transcapitotriquetral perilunate fracture-dislocation patterns do occur, but little has been reported regarding their treatment. An understanding of the pathomechanics, patterns of injury, radiographic findings, and outcomes involved can assist in the management of these injuries.

CLASSIFICATION

Perilunate injuries result from excessive forces applied to the dorsiflexed wrist with significant dorsal compression and anterior tension. The mechanisms of injury as described by Mayfield and associates[1] are the basis of current understanding of these injuries. Mayfield and associates described four stages of injury occurring about the lunate: stage I, scapholunate disruption; stage II, dorsal displacement of the capitate; stage III, lunotriquetral disruption; and stage IV, lunate dislocation. The addition of radial or ulnar deviation results in distinct patterns of injury, with the severity of injury proportional to the applied force.[2] Fractures of the bones surrounding the lunate occur prior to the dislocation of the lunate and depend on the position of the wrist, the direction of the applied force, and the contraction of the muscles and tendons that cross the wrist.

The concept of lesser arc and greater arc injuries was introduced by Johnson[3] in 1980 (Fig. 1). He defined lesser arc injuries as purely ligamentous disruptions, following the mechanism outlined by Mayfield and associates, and greater arc injuries as injuries that involve disruptions of the osseous structures surrounding the lunate.

In 1980, Green and O'Brien[4] developed a classification of carpal dislocations that organizes dislocations into six major types based on their clinical management (Table 1). This system was based on the presence of a subluxated or fractured scaphoid and the direction of displacement of the distal carpal row. The perilunate dislocations involving the capitate and triquetrum include types IVB, IVC, and IVD.

TABLE 1

Classification of Carpal Dislocations

Type I	Dorsal perilunate dislocation
Type II	Transscaphoid perilunate fracture-dislocation
Type III	Palmar dislocation
Type IV	Variants
IVA	Transradial styloid perilunate dislocation
IVB	Naviculocapitate syndrome
IVC	Transtriquetral fracture-dislocation
IVD	Types that defy classification
Type V	Injuries with an isolated rotary scaphoid subluxation
Type VI	Total dislocations of the scaphoid

FIGURE 1

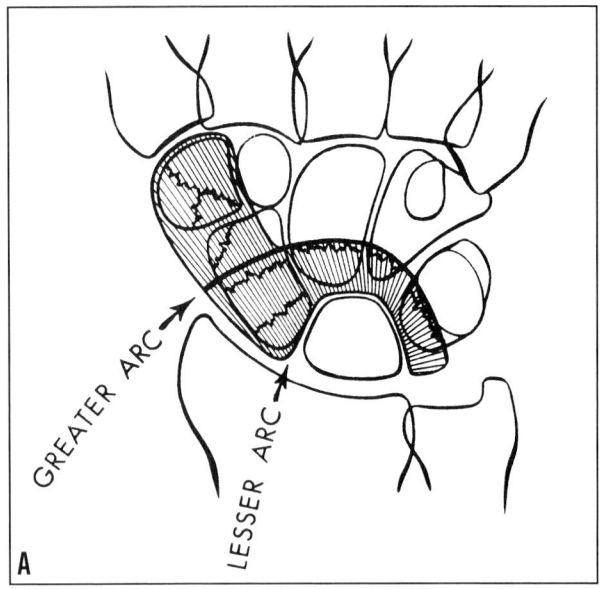

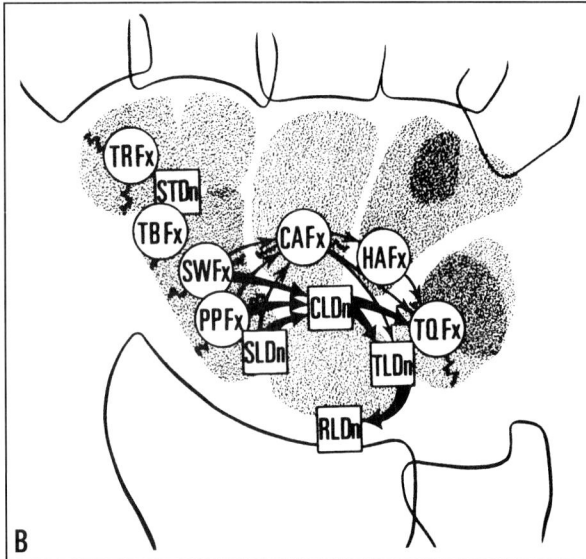

The pathways of ligamentous and bone injury about the wrist. **A,** The lesser arc injuries represent the ligamentous disruptions that were described by Mayfield and associates. **B,** Greater arc injuries are those that occur through the carpal bones. The circles represent fractures, and the boxes represent dislocations. TRFx = trapezial fracture; STDn = scaphotrapezial dislocation; TBFx = tuberosity fracture; SWFx = scaphoid waist fracture; PPFx = proximal-pole fracture; SLDn = scapholunate dislocation; CAFx = capitate fracture; CLDn = capitolunate dislocation; HAFx = hamate fracture; TQFx = triquetral fracture; TLDn = triquetro-lunate dislocation; RLDn = radiolunate dislocation; SWFx + CAFx + HAFx + TQFx = greater arc injuries; SLDn + CLDn + TLDn = lesser arc injuries. (Reproduced with permission from Johnson RP: The acutely injured wrist and its residuals. *Clin Orthop* 1980;149:33-44.)

TRANSSCAPHOID, TRANSCAPITATE PERILUNATE INJURIES

Perves and associates[5] were the first to describe a transscaphoid, transcapitate perilunate fracture-dislocation, in 1937. Nearly 20 years later, Fenton[6] described a similar fracture pattern and introduced the term scaphocapitate or naviculocapitate syndrome (Fig. 2). Fenton described two patients, each of whom sustained a proximal capitate fracture that was rotated 180° after a fall on an outstretched hand. Neither of Fenton's patients was reported to have an associated perilunate dislocation, which led to great confusion because most scaphocapitate syndromes subsequently reported have been associated with perilunate dislocations.[7] Some authors have theorized that scaphocapitate syndrome results from a spontaneously reduced transscaphoid, transcapitate perilunate fracture-dislocation.[8]

Mechanism of Injury

Situated in the middle of the carpus, the capitate is surrounded and reinforced by the other carpal bones and ligaments and is not typically subject to fracture.[6,9,10] The capitate is entirely articular, with the exception of vascular foramina located in the neck and waist.[7,11] The intrinsic vascular supply of the capitate originates from the middle third of the bone and is without a collateral supply.[12] The unique architecture of its foramina and intrinsic vascular pattern add to the susceptibility of fracture and progression to nonunion or osteonecrosis. Although high-energy trauma is the norm,[13-15] in Adler and Shaftan's review of 91 capitate fractures,[9] indirect trauma was the most common mechanism of fracture of the capitate. The capitate fracture results from direct impact against the dorsal radius with the wrist hyperextended and deviated ulnarly.[14,16] If the wrist continues to hyperextend, the proximal fragment rotates 90°. As the wrist returns to neutral, the distal fragment may again rotate to 180° from its original position.[16,17] Although the most common pattern of rotation of the proximal pole of the capitate is 180°, it may be limited to only 90° of rotation, depending on the degree of insult.[13] Furthermore, other osseous structures may be damaged; case reports have described scaphocapitate syndrome with a concomitant radial styloid fracture.[14,18]

Diagnosis

Although routine radiographs are requisite in the evaluation of wrist fracture-dislocations, traction radiographs

FIGURE 2

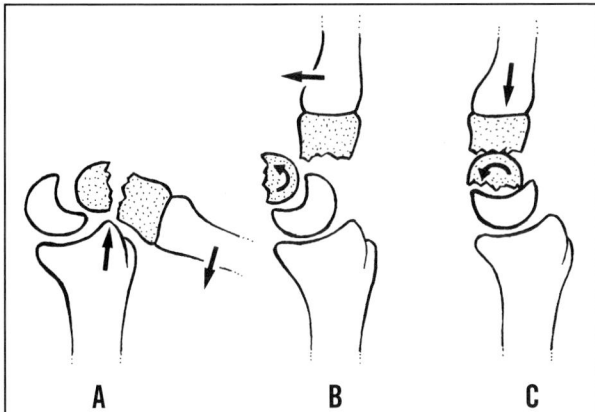

The mechanism by which the fracture-dislocation of the capitate occurs as part of the scaphocapitate syndrome as first proposed by Fenton. **A,** Extreme wrist hyperextension results in an impaction of the neck of the capitate against the dorsal radius, resulting in a transverse proximal capitate fracture. **B,** When the wrist is brought back to neutral, the roughened fracture surface results in greater displacement of the unconstrained proximal capitate fracture. **C,** The subsequent axial compression results in further displacement and a fracture fragment that has rotated 180°. (Reproduced with permission from Garcia-Elias M: Carpal instabilities and dislocations, in Green DP, Hotchkiss RN, Pederson WC (eds): *Green's Operative Hand Surgery*, ed 4. New York, NY, Churchill Livingstone, 1999, pp 865-928.)

at time of reduction are recommended, as they often assist in the assessment of ligament and osseous injury.[17] The squared-off proximal portion of the capitate usually can be easily seen and has been described as having a "cut-off-top-of-an-egg" appearance[15] (Fig. 3). The transscaphoid, transcapitate perilunate fracture-dislocation can be overlooked even if complete sets of radiographs are taken, especially if the dislocation reduces spontaneously. Boisgard and associates[19] reported on 26 cases, of which eight were unrecognized at presentation despite adequate radiographs. CT is often helpful in the diagnosis of scaphocapitate syndrome.[20]

Treatment

In 1955, Jones[21] reported the treatment of a patient with scaphocapitate syndrome by immobilization only. The capitate was allowed to heal with the proximal portion rotated 180°. The results were reported as excellent, and the resultant range of motion was "three-quarters of the normal wrist."[21] Adler and Shaftan[9] described healing of the capitate in the malrotated position, in addition to osteonecrosis of both the scaphoid and capitate. The

FIGURE 3

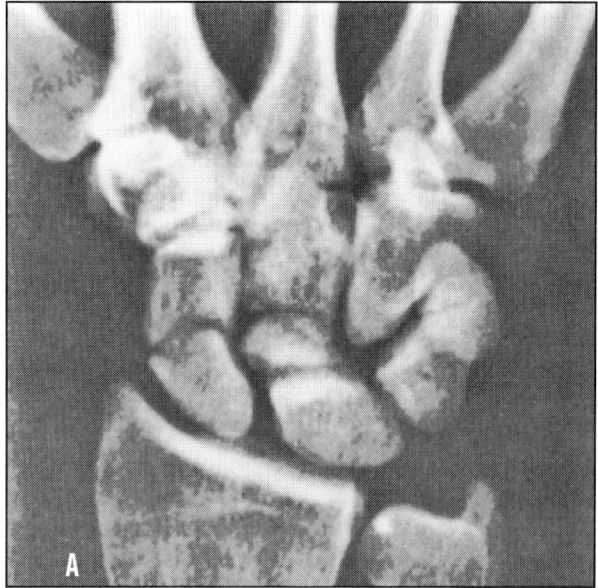

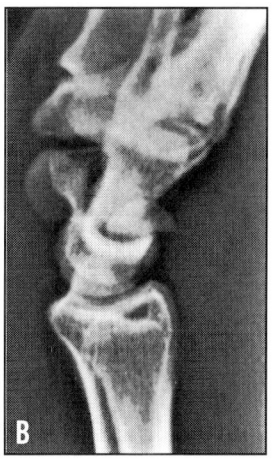
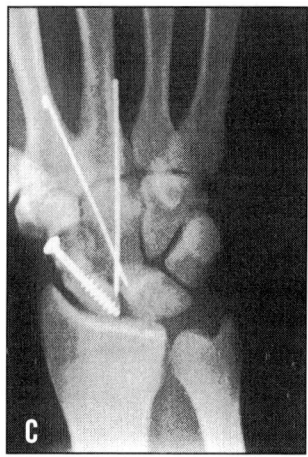

A transscaphoid, transcapitate perilunate fracture-dislocation, also known as naviculocapitate or scaphocapitate syndrome. AP **(A)** and lateral **(B)** radiographs show the characteristic "cut-off-top-of-an-egg" appearance, which results from the 180°-rotated proximal capitate fragment. (Reproduced with permission from Meyers MH, Wells R, Harvey JP Jr: Naviculo-capitate fracture syndrome: Review of the literature and a case report. *J Bone Joint Surg Am* 1971;53:1383-1386.) **C,** Surgical management of these injuries included anatomic and rigid fixation of the scaphoid and capitate fractures. (Reproduced with permission from Dinesh MKS, Sukul K, Johannes EJ: Transscapho-transcapitate fracture-dislocation of the carpus. *J Hand Surg Am* 1992;17:348-353.)

patient had painless range of motion and full function at follow-up 8 months later.[9] In yet another report, Marsh and Lampros[10] described a patient in whom the scaphocapitate syndrome was missed at presentation; follow-up

FIGURE 4

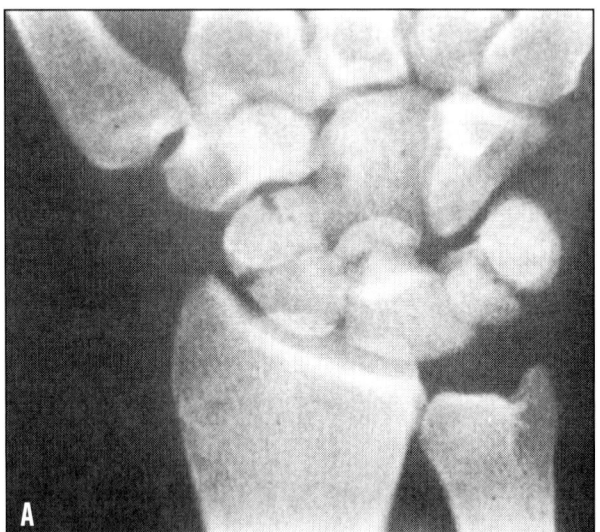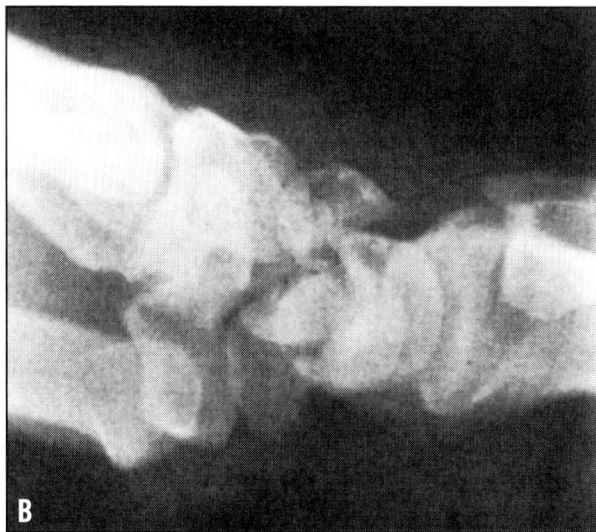

A transscaphoid, transcapitate, transtriquetral perilunate injury. **A,** AP radiograph. **B,** Lateral radiograph. (Reproduced with permission from Cooney WP, Bussey R, Dobyns JH, Linscheid RL: Difficult wrist fractures: Perilunate fracture-dislocations of the wrist. *Clin Orthop* 1987;214:136-147.)

revealed an asymptomatic osteonecrosis of the proximal pole of the scaphoid.

Several authors have advocated excision of the proximal pole of the capitate.[6,14] Fenton[6] reported that this was easily accomplished and believed that osteonecrosis and nonunion of the capitate were inevitable. Nicholson[8] attempted open reduction of this type of injury but later stated that excision may have been wiser. Others have recommended primary arthrodesis when anatomic reduction could not be obtained by closed methods.[22]

In contrast to these earlier results, more recent reports have demonstrated that symptomatic capitate necrosis and nonunion are common with nonsurgical treatment, whereas long-term results have been invariably good with early open reduction and internal fixation.[19] Multiple authors have reported on open reduction via a dorsal or palmar approach and fixation of the capitate with Kirschner wires (K-wires) or screws.[7,15,19,23,24] In these series, all capitate fractures healed between 2 and 6 months after surgery. Once anatomic reduction and fixation of the capitate fragment is achieved, transient avascular changes in the proximal pole of the capitate are common; however, healing typically occurs.[17] Furthermore, the capitate fragment, once replaced to its original position, ensures correct ligament tension and stability.[25]

Surgical treatment with the goal of anatomic restoration must be the primary objective in the treatment of transscaphoid, transcapitate perilunate fracture-dislocations. Any loss of alignment in the carpus will lead to incongruity and, eventually, degenerative arthritis. The concern that surgical reduction might lead to necrosis of the head of the capitate is unjustified.[13]

The first step in surgical treatment is the reduction and fixation of the capitate fracture.[23] If this is not performed initially, the distal fragment of the scaphoid tends to migrate medially, making its reduction and stabilization difficult. In cases where the capitate is comminuted, primary bone grafting may be indicated.[26]

When scaphocapitate syndrome is associated with a radial styloid fracture, the surgical treatment described in the literature has varied.[14,18] In the two cases reported, one patient was treated with immobilization, the other with open reduction and internal fixation. In the patient treated nonsurgically, the proximal fragment of the capitate was eventually excised, and osteonecrosis ensued.[14] In the other patient, open reduction and fixation of the capitate fragment, scaphoid, and radial styloid fractures was performed. Despite slight posttraumatic arthritis, the loss of function was minimal, and the patient returned to work.[18] These cases illustrate the importance of anatomic restoration to achieve optimal outcome.

Treatment after nonunion or osteonecrosis of the capitate or scaphoid is directed at relieving pain and salvaging motion and function if possible. Scaphoid and lunate excision have been reported, with uniformly poor outcomes.[15,27]

FIGURE 5

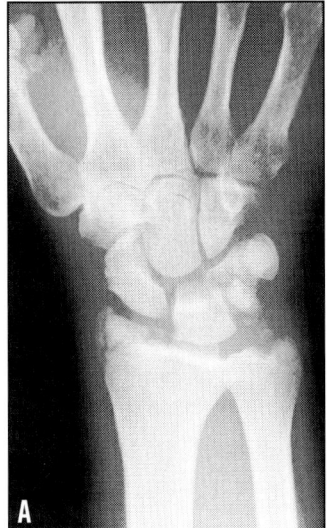 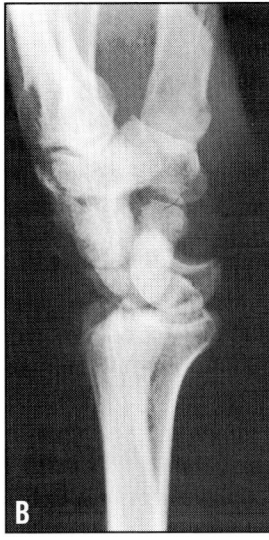 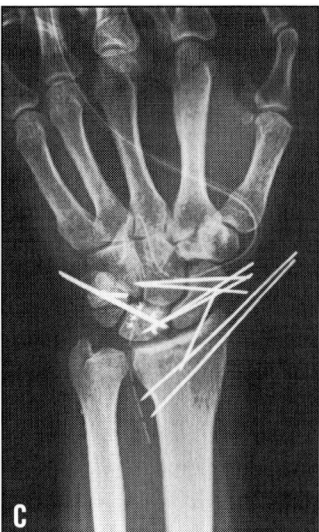 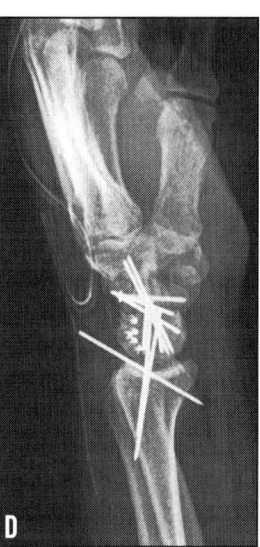

A transradial styloid, transtriquetral perilunate fracture-dislocation. **A,** AP radiograph. **B,** Lateral radiograph. **C** and **D,** Surgical management included rigid fixation of the body fracture of the triquetrum with repair of the avulsed lunotriquetral ligament and bone fragment back to the triquetrum, in addition to repair of the scapholunate ligament and palmar closure of the space of Poirier.

Although a proximal row carpectomy is an option for delayed or salvage treatment,[28] lack of articular cartilage and necrosis of the proximal capitate often preclude this option. When significant cartilage damage is present, or in cases in which reduction cannot be accomplished, total wrist arthrodesis may be indicated.[29]

Few long-term follow-up studies of scaphocapitate syndrome exist; however, some patients have reportedly returned to demanding manual labor. Despite this, patients should be advised that late sequelae, including degenerative arthritis, are the norm.[13]

TRANSSCAPHOID, TRANSCAPITATE, TRANSTRIQUETRAL PERILUNATE INJURIES

The transscaphoid, transcapitate, transtriquetral perilunate injuries represent the only true greater arc injuries and are exceedingly rare. A thorough review of the literature has identified only three cases of this injury. In the first case, reported in 1959, the injury was not recognized at presentation.[10] This injury was treated with immobilization, despite the 180°-rotated capitate fracture. The triquetral avulsion, as well as an associated ulnar styloid fracture, was reported as reduced with early healing, whereas the capitate demonstrated osteonecrosis. No long-term follow-up was reported.

The second report involved a 19-year-old man who sustained a fall of approximately 9 feet.[26] In addition to a comminuted fracture of the midshaft ipsilateral humerus, radiographs showed a transscaphoid, transcapitate, transtriquetral perilunate dislocation (Fig. 4). After closed reduction, the transcapitate fracture was recognized and found to be displaced. Open reduction, internal fixation, and bone grafting of the capitate and scaphoid ensued; the triquetrum was not treated. Anatomic reduction was reported, and all fractures united by 13 weeks. By 6 months the patient was asymptomatic and lacked only the extremes of wrist flexion and extension. At 2-year follow-up, radiographs demonstrated complete healing without osteonecrosis.

In the third patient, anatomic restoration of the fractures was accomplished with screw fixation of the capitate after reduction. At 10-week follow-up, the patient had minimal pain, good strength, consolidation of the scaphoid and triquetrum, and incomplete healing of the capitate.[30]

In these three cases, the treatment, diagnosis, and outcome of transscaphoid, transcapitate, transtriquetral perilunate injuries were similar to those for the scaphocapitate or naviculocapitate syndrome. If fractured, the capitate is often rotated, and if it is left unreduced, it will progress to osteonecrosis. However, early open reduction and fixation often leads to good to excellent outcomes.

Additionally, although in all cases the triquetral fracture was not specifically treated, the fracture reduced with reduction of the dislocation and progressed to union.

TRANSTRIQUETRAL PERILUNATE INJURIES

As previously mentioned, the triquetrum may fracture in association with the capitate, scaphoid, radial styloid, or some combination thereof. However, in some carpal dislocations, the line of cleavage may be purely ligamentous except for extension through the triquetrum. An injury to the lunotriquetral joint may cause a palmar-to-dorsal rupture or avulsion of the intervening ligament. Approximately one quarter of these injuries include a sagittal fracture of either the body or a proximal pole of the triquetrum.[31] The proximal pole stays attached to the lunate via the intact lunotriquetral ligament, allowing for the proximal pole to displace with the capitate. This fragment may be a single large bony fragment or may be severely comminuted (Fig. 5).

Some authors believe that reduction of the midcarpal joint restores the triquetral fracture to an acceptable position; they therefore pay little attention to this fracture except for removing nonviable bone fragments.[4] In one series of 47 perilunate fracture-dislocations, triquetral fractures occurred in only four. However, the authors made no specific recommendations with regard to the treatment of these injuries.[32] Cooney and associates[2] treated transtriquetral fractures with multiple K-wires. Caution must be taken to prevent malrotation of the triquetrum. Labbe and associates[25] reported that these fractures should not be excised but carefully replaced in their original position at the time of an open procedure. Skelly and associates[33] described an unusual palmar lunate transtriquetral fracture-dislocation. After attempted closed reduction, the fragment was thought to be reduced. The wrist required an open reduction because of persistent scapholunate dissociation, and at that time it was noted that the articular surface of the proximal triquetral fragment was rotated 180° on its transverse axis. It was necessary to rotate and reduce the triquetral fragment before obtaining complete anatomic reduction of the scapholunate interval. Reduction could be achieved only by derotating the fragment and "untwisting" the lunotriquetral ligament. The authors speculated that traction radiographs at the time of reduction likely would have revealed the rotated proximal triquetral fragment.

TRANSSCAPHOID, TRANSTRIQUETRAL PERILUNATE INJURIES

Variants of the transscaphoid perilunate dislocation include those that are associated with fractures of the triquetrum. Although these injuries are rarely separated, they do deserve special mention. Many reports discuss in detail the treatment of the scaphoid but fail to address treatment required for the triquetral fracture.

Various treatments have been described for transscaphoid perilunate dislocations associated with a fracture of the triquetrum. Campbell and associates[34] reported on a patient with this same pattern but also a dorsal dislocation. The injury was treated by open reduction and fixation of the triquetrum with K-wires. However, because of the comminution of the triquetral fracture, anatomic restoration was unsuccessful. Once the lunate and scaphoid were reduced, the large fragment of triquetrum was restored to its anatomic position. In another patient with transscaphoid, transtriquetral palmar lunate dislocation, open reduction could not be achieved; therefore, a proximal row carpectomy was performed.[35]

In a series of transscaphoid perilunate fracture-dislocations in which four of the 17 cases demonstrated triquetral fractures, no treatment of the triquetral fractures was described except for closed reduction.[36] All wrists were treated with open reduction and fixation of the scaphoid. At an average follow-up of 2.7 years, the scaphoid had healed in 15 of the 17 wrists. From the overall good results as indicated by symptoms, clinical examination, and radiographs, it can be assumed that most if not all the triquetral fractures had healed.

INJURIES INVOLVING FRACTURE OF THE TRANSRADIAL STYLOID

The literature includes one case of a transscaphoid, transtriquetral perilunate injury with an added transradial styloid fracture. Closed reduction was unsuccessful, so open reduction and internal fixation with a Herbert screw via a Russe approach was performed on the scaphoid fracture, followed by reduction and percutaneous pinning of the radial styloid. No attempt was made to restore the triquetrum. K-wires and immobilization were discontinued at 6 weeks, and 1 year postoperatively the scaphoid and radial styloid had united, but the avulsion fracture of the triquetrum had not. The patient experienced no wrist discomfort, however, and had returned to work. His wrist functional score was consistent with good function.[37]

Another variation, a transradial styloid, transtriquetral perilunate injury with an associated fracture of the ulnar border of the distal radius, was described.[38] Acute reduction of the perilunate dislocation and the triquetral fracture was performed under intravenous analgesia. Treatment of the distal radius fracture consisted of open reduction with pinning in addition to external fixation. Although at 1 year the patient was able to return to work, the associated ulnar styloid fracture had not achieved union and the patient had unsatisfactory wrist function.[38]

Two further possible variations include a transradial styloid, transcapitate, transtriquetral perilunate injury and a transradial styloid, transscaphoid, transcapitate, transtriquetral perilunate injury. Such injuries have not yet been reported in the literature to our knowledge.

Conclusion

The relative rarity of perilunate fracture-dislocations involving the capitate or triquetrum makes determination of a preferred treatment method based on evidence-based clinical series difficult if not impossible. However, in reviewing the many available case reports and series, it is apparent that most authors recommend at minimum the anatomic restoration of the scaphoid fracture without addressing the other concomitant fractures. However, treatment cannot be guided by the fracture pattern alone without consideration of the concomitant soft-tissue injuries.

Based on previous studies of intra-articular fractures and the multiple case reports of the many variants of perilunate fracture-dislocations that involve the capitate and triquetrum, the goals of reconstructive surgery should be twofold. The first goal is anatomic restoration of fractures, while the second is the repair or reconstruction of soft-tissue injuries.

A high degree of suspicion and careful review of radiographs will often identify these rare perilunate fracture-dislocation variants. Once identified, reconstruction based on the principles of anatomic restoration of osseous and soft-tissue elements will achieve the optimal outcome.

References

1. Mayfield JK, Johnson RP, Kilcoyne RK: Carpal dislocations: Pathomechanics and progressive perilunar instability. *J Hand Surg Am* 1980;5:226-241.

2. Cooney WP, Bussey R, Dobyns JH, Linscheid RL: Difficult wrist fractures: Perilunate fracture-dislocations of the wrist. *Clin Orthop* 1987;214:136-147.

3. Johnson RP: The acutely injured wrist and its residuals. *Clin Orthop* 1980;149:33-44.

4. Green DP, O'Brien ET: Classification and management of carpal dislocations. *Clin Orthop* 1980;149:55-72.

5. Perves J, Rigaud A, Badelon L: Fracture par decapitation du grand os avec deplacement dorsal du corps de los simulant une dislocation carpienne. *Rev d' Orthop* 1937;24: 251-253.

6. Fenton RL: The naviculo-capitate fracture syndrome. *J Bone Joint Surg Am* 1956;38:681-684.

7. Meyers MH, Wells R, Harvey JP Jr: Naviculo-capitate fracture syndrome: Review of the literature and a case report. *J Bone Joint Surg Am* 1971;53:1383-1386.

8. Nicholson CB: Fracture dislocation of the os magnum. *J R Nav Med Serv* 1940;26:289-291.

9. Adler JB, Shaftan GW: Fractures of the capitate. *J Bone Joint Surg Am* 1962;44:1537-1547.

10. Marsh AP, Lampros PJ: The naviculo-capitate fracture syndrome. *AJR Am J Roentgenol Radium Ther Nucl Med* 1959;82:255-256.

11. Kaplan EB (ed): *Functional and Surgical Anatomy of the Hand.* Philadelphia, PA, JB Lippincott, 1953.

12. Barber H: The intraosseous and arterial anatomy of the adult human carpus. *Orthop Oxford* 1972;3:1-20.

13. Kaulesar Sukul DM, Johannes EJ: Transscapho-transcapitate fracture dislocation of the carpus. *J Hand Surg Am* 1992;17:348-353.

14. Stein F, Siegel MW: Naviculocapitate fracture syndrome: A case report: New thoughts on the mechanism of injury. *J Bone Joint Surg Am* 1969;51:391-395.

15. Ipsen T, Larsen CF: A case of scapho-capitate fracture. *Acta Orthop Scand* 1985;56:509-510.

16. Monahan PR, Galasko CS: The scapho-capitate fracture syndrome: A mechanism of injury. *J Bone Joint Surg Br* 1972;54:122-124.

17. Garcia-Elias M: Carpal instabilities and dislocations, in Green DP, Hotchkiss RN, Pederson WC (eds): *Green's Operative Hand Surgery,* ed 4. New York, NY, Churchill Livingstone, 1999, pp 909-928.

18. Pfeiffer KM: Perilunar, transscaphoid, transcapital, transstyloid fracture-dislocation of the wrist: Operative reconstruction. *Handchir* 1978;10:39-40.

19. Boisgard S, Bremont JL, Guyonnet G, Chatenet T, Levai JP: Scapho-capitate fracture: Apropos of a case, review of the literature. *Ann Chir Main Memb Super* 1996;15: 181-188.

20. Moneim MS: Management of greater arc carpal fractures. *Hand Clin* 1988;4:457-467.

21. Jones GB: An unusual fracture-dislocation of the carpus. *J Bone Joint Surg Br* 1955;37:146-147.

22. Wagner CJ: Perilunar dislocations. *J Bone Joint Surg Am* 1956;38:1198-1207.

23. Vance RM, Gelberman RH, Evans EF: Scaphocapitate fractures: Patterns of dislocation, mechanisms of injury, and preliminary results of treatment. *J Bone Joint Surg Am* 1980;62:271-276.

24. El-Khoury GY, Usta HY, Blair WF: Naviculocapitate fracture-dislocation. *AJR Am J Roentgenol* 1982;139:385-386.

25. Labbe JL, Vachaud M, Rouge D, Ficat P: Trans-scapho-perilunar dislocations with internal instability of the carpal bones. *Rev Chir Orthop Reparatrice Appar Mot* 1986;72:53-62.

26. Weseley MS, Barenfeld PA: Trans-scaphoid, transcapitate, transtriquetral, perilunate fracture-dislocation of the wrist: A case report. *J Bone Joint Surg Am* 1972;54:1073-1078.

27. Cave EF: Retrolunar dislocation of the capitate with fracture or subluxation of the navicular bone. *J Bone Joint Surg Am* 1941;23:830-840.

28. Inoue G, Miura T: Proximal row carpectomy in perilunate dislocations and lunatomalacia. *Acta Orthop Scand* 1990;61:449-452.

29. Hastings DE, Silver RL: Intercarpal arthrodesis in the management of chronic carpal instability after trauma. *J Hand Surg Am* 1984;9:834-840.

30. Hohenbleicher R: The "naviculo-capitate fracture" syndrome. *Unfallheilkunde* 1976;79:281-283.

31. Garcia-Elias M, Irisarri C, Henriquez A, et al: Perilunar dislocation of the carpus: A diagnosis still often missed. *Ann Chir Main* 1986;5:281-287.

32. Russell TB: Inter-carpal dislocations and fracture-dislocations: A review of fifty-nine cases. *J Bone Joint Surg Br* 1949;31:524-531.

33. Skelly WJ, Nahigian SH, Hidvegi EB: Palmar lunate transtriquetral fracture-dislocation. *J Hand Surg Am* 1991;16:536-539.

34. Campbell RD Jr, Thompson TC, Lance EM, Adler JB: Indications for open reduction of lunate and perilunate dislocations of the carpal bones. *J Bone Joint Surg Am* 1965;47:915-937.

35. Woodward AH, Neviaser RJ, Nisenfeld F: Radial and volar perilunate transscaphoid fracture dislocation. *South Med J* 1975;68:926-928.

36. Moneim MS, Hofammann KE III, Omer GE: Trans-scaphoid perilunate fracture-dislocation: Result of open reduction and pin fixation. *Clin Orthop* 1984;190:227-235.

37. Schranz PJ, Fagg PS: Trans-radial styloid, trans-scaphoid, trans-triquetral perilunate dislocation. *J R Army Med Corps* 1991;137:146-148.

38. Yamaguchi H, Takahara M: Transradial styloid, transtriquetral perilunate dislocation of the carpus with an associated fracture of the ulnar border of the distal radius. *J Orthop Trauma* 1994;8:434-436.

CHAPTER 8

LATE MANAGEMENT OF PERILUNATE FRACTURE-DISLOCATIONS

MATTHEW M. TOMAINO, MD

Optimal outcome following acute perilunate fracture-dislocations requires accurate restoration of carpal alignment as well as fracture stabilization and union for greater arc injuries and satisfactory reduction and ligamentous healing for lesser arc injuries. These injuries are so severe, however, that even if the foregoing conditions are met, the patient may experience substantial loss of wrist motion and grip strength,[1-3] residual carpal instability, and painful scapholunate advanced collapse (SLAC) arthritis.[4]

Early diagnosis and accurate open reduction and stabilization of perilunate fracture-dislocations are associated with improved outcome;[1,5] however, these injuries are missed as much as 25% of the time.[1] Unfortunately, the outcome appears to deteriorate when treatment is delayed longer than 1 week.[1,6]

This chapter addresses the late management of perilunate fracture-dislocations. It discusses both neglected (chronic) injuries and, briefly, those for which adequate early treatment has been complicated by carpal instability, osteonecrosis, nonunion, or SLAC arthritis.

CHRONIC PERILUNATE FRACTURE-DISLOCATIONS

Presentation

The literature indicates two reasons that early diagnosis of perilunate fracture-dislocations may be missed: (1) The patient views the wrist injury as a benign sprain and does not seek evaluation; (2) More commonly, the physician interprets the radiographs incorrectly because the overlapping carpal bones present a challenge to those unfamiliar with radiographic anatomy. Few reports specifically address the late treatment of neglected injuries;[7-13] most of those that do are either case reports or involve a small number of patients.

Incapacitating wrist pain, weakness, and limited motion often prompt patients with perilunate fracture-dislocations to seek medical attention eventually. Paresthesias are common, particularly with palmar lunate or perilunate dislocations. Despite the severity of these injuries, however, subjective complaints may be limited to the symptoms of carpal tunnel syndrome. Siegert and associates[10] reported on two patients who presented 42 and 53 years after injury because of worsening paresthesias.[9] Similarly, I diagnosed a chronic dorsal perilunate dislocation in an 88-year-old woman 60 years after she allegedly fell on an outstretched hand (Fig. 1). Her only symptoms were worsening median nerve distribution paresthesias and numbness; her 40° arc of wrist motion was pain free.

Treatment

The following treatment options have been described in the literature: (1) open reduction and internal fixation (ORIF), (2) proximal row carpectomy (PRC), (3) wrist fusion, (4) isolated carpal bone excision, and (5) carpal tunnel release. Both patient-related and injury-related variables influence decision making. These include symptoms (or lack thereof), an assessment of functional impairment, length of time since the injury, the status of articular cartilage, the presence of arthritis or osteonecrosis, and underlying injury pattern (greater arc or lesser arc).

Wrist scores should not be used alone to assess outcome following treatment of these neglected fracture-dislocations. Patient satisfaction revolves around pain relief more often than grip strength or range of motion.[14] Indeed, functional range of motion requires only 5° of wrist flex-

FIGURE 1

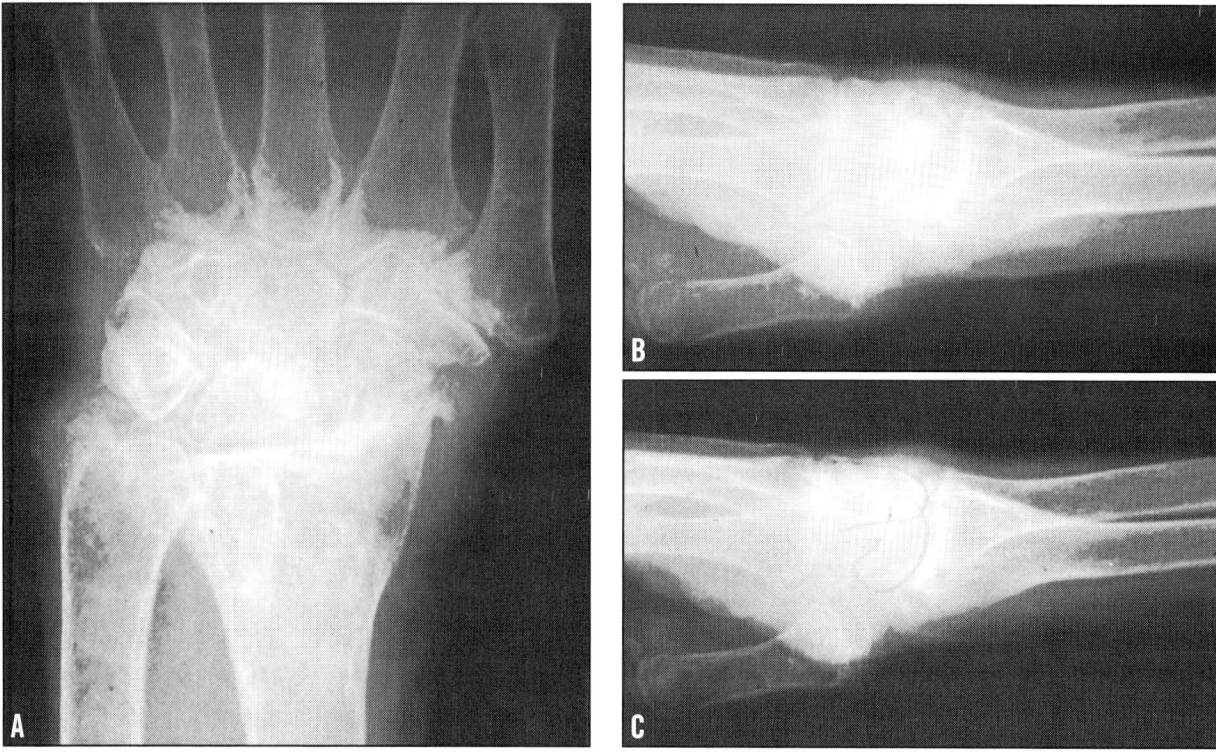

Radiographs of the wrist of an 88-year-old patient who presented with worsening paresthesias and numbness but no wrist pain or impaired grip strength. Both the PA radiograph **(A)** and lateral radiographs **(B,C)** show a chronic perilunate dislocation with radioscaphoid and intercarpal arthritis. The patient was completely satisfied with the outcome following carpal tunnel release alone.

ion and 30° of extension.[15] When assessing results, therefore, pain relief is perhaps the most critical parameter.

Open Reduction and Internal Fixation Several authors[7,9-12] have provided anecdotal support for the use of ORIF in perilunate fracture-dislocations. Vegter[8] described the use of gradual distraction with an external fixator to restore carpal height and facilitate "semi-closed" reduction in two patients. Beginning 5 and 6 weeks following missed palmar dislocation of the lunate, slight distraction was maintained for 6 weeks, until fixator removal. Final review was performed at only 5 and 6 months, respectively, and the quality of the outcome from the patient's perspective was not mentioned. Mizuseki and associates (unpublished data, third combined meeting of the Japanese and American Societies for Surgery of the Hand, Maui, Hawaii, 2000) acknowledged the challenges of open reduction because of scar formation and soft-tissue contracture. They described successful reduction performed in three patients an average of 19 weeks following injury, but one injury was nearly 33 weeks old. The

technique included the placement of two pins in the second metacarpal and two in the radius. The radiocarpal joint was distracted 5 to 7 mm, such that the capitate was level with the dorsal edge of the lunate, within 7 to 14 days of the initiation of distraction. At that time a dorsal surgical approach allowed reduction and stabilization with Kirschner wires (K-wires), which were left in place for 4 to 5 weeks. At an average follow-up of 5½ years, the authors found an average improvement in grip strength of 17 kg and an improvement in flexion and extension of 28° and 25°. The authors did not provide information regarding patient satisfaction. Intercarpal arthritis was noted radiographically in one wrist.

More traditional open reduction surgery has used both dorsal and combined palmar and dorsal approaches (Fig. 2). The latter is mandatory in the setting of concomitant carpal tunnel syndrome and palmar lunate dislocation. No definitive statement regarding the effect of the length of delay on the outcome of treatment is possible because of the small number of cases treated by ORIF. Seven weeks

FIGURE 2

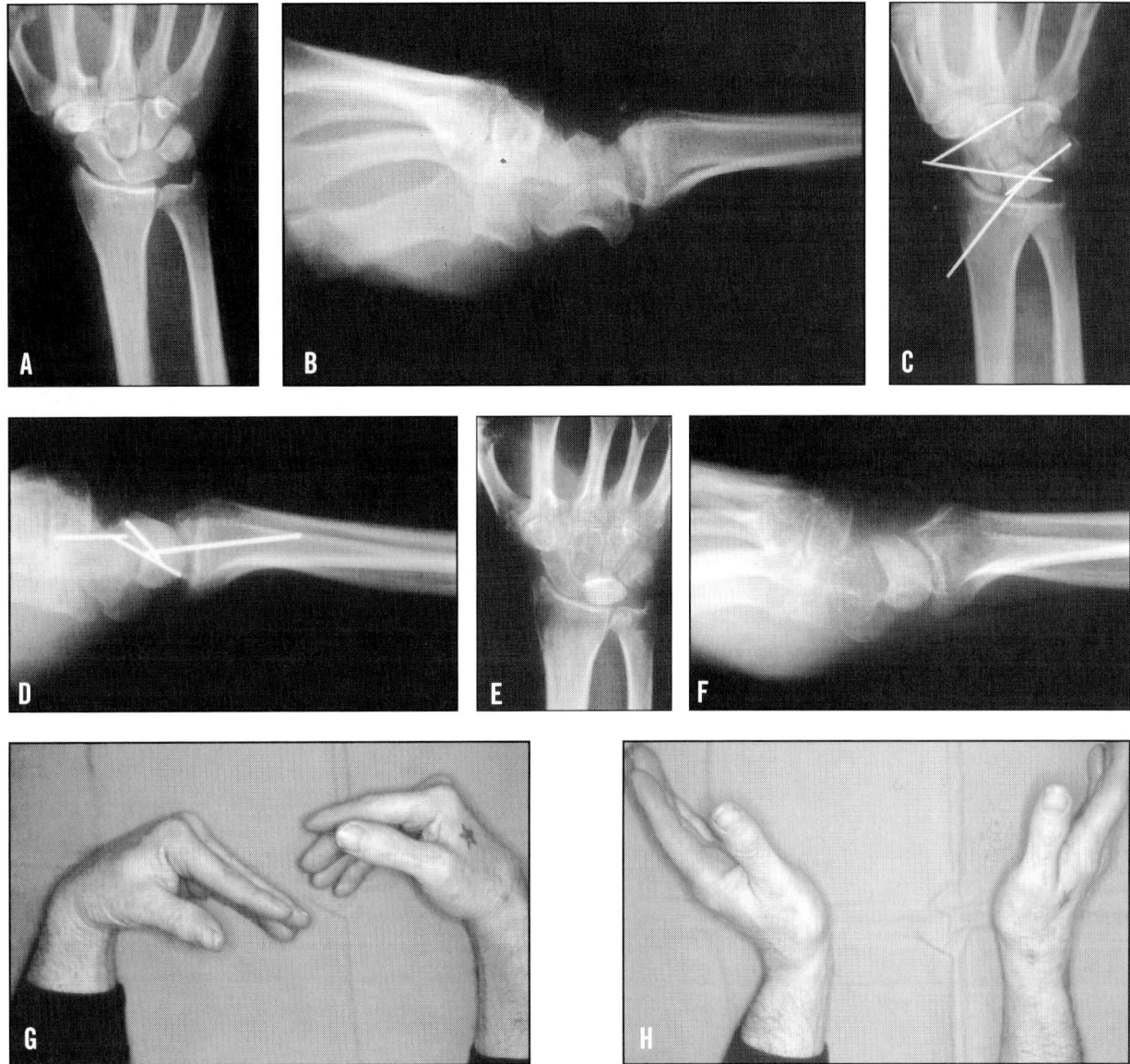

Treatment of neglected palmar lunate dislocation. PA **(A)** and lateral **(B)** radiographs show the wrist 6 weeks after injury. PA **(C)** and lateral **(D)** radiographs show restored intercarpal relationships following ORIF using a combined dorsal and palmar approach. PA **(E)** and lateral **(F)** radiographs show the same wrist 18 months following surgery. Osteonecrosis of the lunate has developed, but there is no evidence of radiocarpal or intercarpal arthritis. Wrist flexion **(G)** and wrist extension **(H)** 18 months following ORIF show a functional arc of motion. The wrist was pain free, and the patient was satisfied with the outcome.

after a palmar lunate dislocation, Howard and Dell[7] performed not only ORIF with K-wires, but also scapholunate ligament reconstruction using a distally based strip of extensor carpi radialis brevis tendon. The authors may have chosen ligament reconstruction because they were pessimistic about the intrinsic healing capacity of the scapholunate ligament. In fact, many regard scapholunate ligament disruptions as chronic after 6 to 12 weeks; failed attempts at repair after this length of time may reflect a failure of biology, not of technical execution. For this reason, the outcome after delayed treatment of a greater arc transscaphoid perilunate dislocation may be better than that following treatment of a purely ligamentous lesser arc injury, although Shah and Jones[16] have shown that scaphoid union rates also decline when treatment is delayed, particularly when nonunion exceeds 5 years.

Inoue and Shionoya[12] performed ORIF using a combined dorsal and palmar approach at an average of 16 weeks (range, 6 to 52 weeks) after injury in six wrists. Internal fixation of the scaphoid with a Herbert screw was done in three wrists. The authors reported three good results, one fair, and two poor, and noted that the three satisfactory results occurred in patients who had surgery within 2 months of injury. Siegert and associates[10] provided similar treatment in six wrists, four with palmar lunate dislocations and two with dorsal perilunate dislocations. The interval between injury and treatment averaged 15 weeks (range, 8 to 35 weeks). In contrast to Inoue and Shionoya, Siegert and associates reported symptomatic improvement at an average follow-up of 3 years in all patients. They concluded that open reduction may yield a satisfactory outcome up to 35 weeks after injury.

Notwithstanding the possibility that external fixation and gradual distraction may facilitate open reduction in cases for which excessive delay results in capsular contracture and scarring, it seems logical that the risk of cartilage damage, secondary arthritis, and osteonecrosis would increase as treatment delay increases (Fig. 2). Transient ischemia of the lunate may occur after perilunate injuries, however, and should not be confused with complete osteonecrosis.[17] In transient ischemia, the palmar wrist ligaments usually remain attached to the dislocated lunate and provide adequate blood supply. Because the ischemia is typically transient, excision of the lunate and possibly even open reduction should be avoided.

Proximal Row Carpectomy In a recent assessment of PRC for chronic perilunate dislocations, Rettig and Raskin[13] acknowledged that delayed ORIF is often unsuccessful because the vascular supply to the carpal bones may be disrupted and soft-tissue contracture may prevent reduction without excessive force and damage to articular cartilage. Rettig and Raskin performed PRC in 12 wrists, each of which had been untreated for a minimum of 8 weeks after injury. They used a combined dorsal and palmar approach, the latter to allow median nerve decompression, lunate excision, and capsuloligamentous repair. Temporary fixation of the radiocapitate joint with a K-wire maintained proper alignment of the wrist during early soft-tissue healing. At an average postoperative fol-

low-up of 40 months, marked relief of wrist pain and improvements in functional motion and grip strength resulted. The average flexion/extension arc was 80°, and grip strength measured 80% of the opposite extremity. Intraoperative evaluation revealed small articular defects in the capitate head in seven wrists. Dorsal capsular interposition was performed in one wrist with capitate degeneration, and at final follow-up the patient was asymptomatic despite radiographic evidence of arthritis.

Siegert and associates[10] performed PRC in two patients, at 47 and 52 weeks after injury. One required secondary radial styloidectomy. At a mean follow-up of 61 months, both patients had unrestricted motion, diminished pain, and improved grip. Inoue and Shionoya[12] performed PRC in 16 wrists through a dorsal approach, at an average of 14 months (range, 2 to 120 months) following injury. In nine patients, the distal pole of the scaphoid was left in place. The authors reported 10 fair and six poor results using a scoring system described by Linscheid and associates.[18] Wrist flexion averaged 31°, wrist extension 39°, radial deviation 5°, and ulnar deviation 24°. The mean flexion/extension arc was 54% of the opposite wrist, and grip strength averaged 63% of the uninjured hand. Although three poor results occurred in wrists in which the articular cartilage of the capitate was worn at the time of surgery, the authors did not comment on whether these patients had satisfactory pain relief. Nor did they provide any information regarding the association between retention of the distal pole of the scaphoid and limited radial deviation.[19]

Notwithstanding relatively few reports in the literature, consensus exists in support of PRC for perilunate fracture-dislocations, even after long delays. A palmar approach may be necessary to perform median nerve decompression; a dorsal approach only is feasible when either carpal tunnel syndrome or palmar lunate dislocation is not present. Integrity of the radioscaphocapitate ligament is required to prevent late ulnar translocation, so surgical repair or temporary radiocapitate pinning may be advisable. Although cartilage damage on the head of the capitate constitutes a traditional contraindication for this procedure, dorsal capsular interposition may allow its use in the late treament of these injuries[19] (Baratz, personal communication, Seattle, Washington, 2000).

Wrist Fusion When significant chondral injury, arthritis, or osteonecrosis contraindicates ORIF or PRC, pancarpal arthrodesis may be the most advisable treatment option for the neglected perilunate fracture-dislocation. Siegert and associates[10] reported successful outcome following arthrodesis 14 weeks after injury in two patients with palmar lunate dislocation. They excised the lunate in both wrists because they appeared avascular, one on radiographs and one during intraoperative inspection. Preliminary PRC may facilitate the technical execution of arthrodesis (radius to distal row) by both decompressing the wrist and removing potentially avascular bones.[20]

Isolated Carpal Bone Excision The few reports of isolated carpal bone excision agree on its lack of success.[10,11] Siegert and associates[10] reported poor results after excision of either the lunate or scaphoid alone in four patients. Similarly, Inoue and Shionoya[11] performed lunate excision through a palmar approach in three patients, accompanied by scaphocapitate arthrodesis in one, and described one fair and three poor results. While scaphocapitate intercarpal arthrodesis and lunate excision have been used in the treatment of Kienböck's disease, this technique does not appear to be a favorable alternative for treating chronic perilunate fracture-dislocations.[5]

Carpal Tunnel Release Carpal tunnel release is clearly indicated in any patient with a neglected perilunate injury when median nerve distribution paresthesias exist. Neurophysiologic confirmation of the diagnosis of carpal tunnel syndrome is probably not necessary, but accurate physical examination is recommended to ensure that there is indeed evidence of nerve sensitivity at the level of the wrist. When numbness and paresthesias accompany lunate dislocation, the diagnosis of carpal tunnel syndrome is unequivocal. In the setting of a dorsal perilunate dislocation, however, it is always worth ruling out potential proximal sources of median nerve distribution irritation, including cervical radiculopathy. When patients report only carpal tunnel–type symptoms, carpal tunnel release alone provides extremely successful treatment (Fig. 1).

My Approach

When chronic perilunate fracture-dislocations are not amenable to ORIF, I consider PRC and midcarpal (four-bone) fusion with scaphoid excision as motion-preserving alternatives to full wrist fusion. Preoperative evaluation of wrist radiographs can be helpful, but I often base my decision between these two options on intraoperative inspection of the proximal pole of the capitate. If capitate arthrosis is present, I prefer four-bone fusion and do not perform a PRC. If lunate fossa arthrosis exists, both motion-preserving options are contraindicated, and I perform full wrist fusion.

Surgical Procedure For either PRC or four-bone fusion, I approach the dorsum of the wrist with a midline incision. I open the retinaculum between the third and fourth compartment and perform a longitudinal capsulotomy. I routinely excise a small segment of posterior interosseous nerve after entering the side of the fourth compartment.

Four-Bone Fusion When capitate arthritis contraindicates PRC, I perform four-bone fusion. I begin by osteotomizing the scaphoid and removing the scaphoid in its entirety. I then use a rongeur to decorticate the adjacent surfaces of the capitate, lunate, triquetrum, and hamate such that adjacent surfaces fit together (Fig. 3). I have been satisfied with both staples and K-wires; when the latter are used, I bury them beneath the skin to minimize the risk of pin tract infections. I place bone graft substitute (usually allograft cancellous bone mixed with commercially available bone matrix proteins) between each of the four decorticated bones before they are aligned and fixated. I immobilize the wrist in a plaster thumb spica cast until the fusion mass is nontender or until radiographic evidence of union develops. This takes from 6 to 10 weeks.

The overwhelming priorities in properly executing four-bone fusion and scaphoid excision include (1) adequate decortication of adjacent surfaces between the lunate and the capitate and between the triquetrum and the hamate; (2) satisfactory bony apposition (scaphoid excision affords the opportunity to ignore the normal intercarpal geome-

FIGURE 3

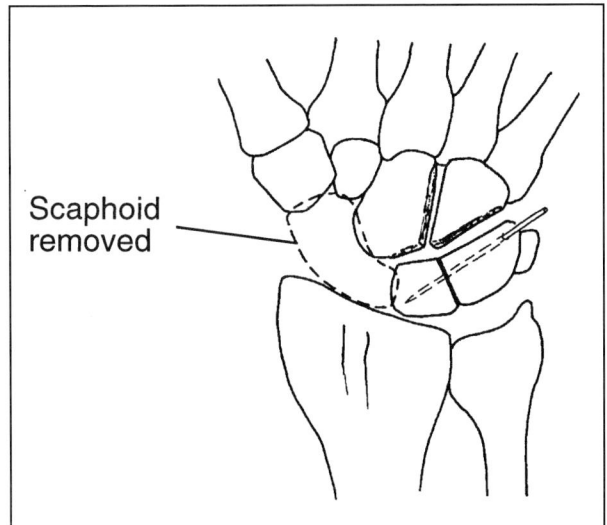

Four-bone fusion with scaphoid excision requires a normal radiolunate joint. Fusion requires adequate decortication and stabilization. (Reproduced with permission from Trumble TE (ed): *Principles of Hand Surgery and Therapy*. Philadelphia, PA, WB Saunders, 2000, p 433.)

FIGURE 4

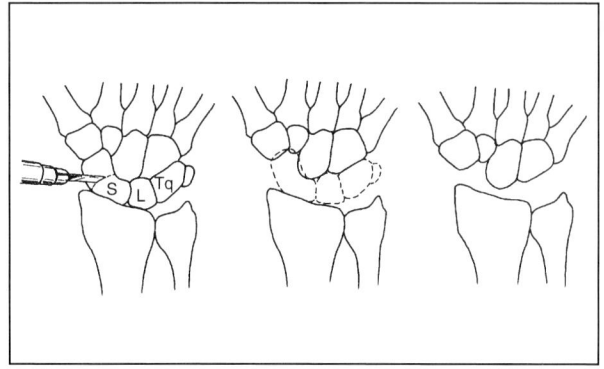

PRC provides a simple hinge joint comprised of a new articulation between the capitate and the lunate fossa. (Reproduced with permission from Trumble TE (ed): *Principles of Hand Surgery and Therapy.* Philadelphia, PA, WB Saunders, 2000, p 434.)

try and achieve bone-bone contact); (3) satisfactory internal fixation, including K-wires, staples, or cannulated screws; (4) correction of lunate extension and restoration of a collinear relationship between capitate and lunate; and (5) adequate postoperative immobilization. If the lunate is not derotated into neutral from its extended position and the capitate is fused in a dorsally subluxated position, as is often present in the wrist with SLAC arthritis, radiocapitate abutment will prevent wrist extension and cause pain. In addition, malalignment of the fused carpal bones—either uncorrected radial translocation of the capitate or residual extension of the lunate—may not completely unload the scaphoid fossa, as CT osteoabsorptiometry has shown.

Although I have achieved greater than 90% union rates using iliac crest and distal radius bone graft, I have switched to bone graft substitutes over the last few years given the small space available for bone graft following decortication and direct capitolunate-triquetrohamate apposition. Bone graft substitutes may be reasonable alternatives to autologous bone, particularly when internal fixation is stable and postoperative immobilization is continued until union is achieved; however, I have noted a decline in union rates to approximately 85% when using these substitutes.

Proximal Row Carpectomy When I perform PRC, I begin by placing K-wire joysticks vertically into the lunate, triquetrum, and scaphoid to facilitate their manipulation when I divide the intercarpal ligaments/or scar tissue. I usually osteotomize the scaphoid at its waist and remove it in its entirety to avoid the potential for impingement

between a retained distal pole and the radial styloid process. Care must be taken during excision of the proximal row not to damage the cartilage of either the proximal pole of the capitate or the lunate fossa. Likewise, care must be taken not to disrupt the radial origin or the intercalary substance of the radioscaphocapitate ligament, which prevents ulnar translocation of the capitate after the procedure. The capitate is allowed to settle into the lunate fossa (Fig. 4). Unless at least 10° of radial deviation is possible without impingement of the trapezoid on the radial styloid process with passive flexion and radial deviation of the wrist, I perform a small radial styloidectomy. After the capsule is closed, the wrist is immobilized for 4 weeks before an active and gentle passive motion program is initiated.

COMPLICATIONS FOLLOWING APPROPRIATE EARLY TREATMENT

Scaphoid nonunion in cases of greater arc injury, ligament incompetence and carpal instability in cases of lesser arc injury, osteonecrosis, and SLAC arthritis are potential long-term complications even when perilunate fracture-dislocations have been treated early and appropriately. Successful management should consider the same variables mentioned previously. Restoration of a pain-free, stable wrist will usually result in high levels of patient satisfaction.[14] Wrist denervation procedures may help, but they are probably not advisable unless preliminary lidocaine infiltration around the anterior and posterior interosseous nerves affords satisfactory pain relief (Berger, unpublished data, Seattle, Washington, 2000). Attempts at salvaging the scaphoid when nonunion complicates transscaphoid perilunate dislocation, or when persistent scapholunate dissociation complicates a lesser arc injury, are likely to be futile because of impaired carpal blood flow, carpal collapse, ligament attrition, and SLAC arthritis.

In these cases, salvage procedures like PRC or four-bone fusion with scaphoid excision are more likely to result in a satisfactory outcome[21] (Fig. 5). Both are contraindicated if radiolunate arthritis exists, however. Four-bone fusion with scaphoid excision is unlikely to succeed in the presence of lunate osteonecrosis, and PRC is relatively contraindicated if significant cartilage damage exists on the head of the capitate. Dorsal capsular interposition may extend the indications for PRC. Wrist arthrodesis also provides effective treatment, but a motion-preserving procedure may be preferred in the absence of contraindications.

FIGURE 5

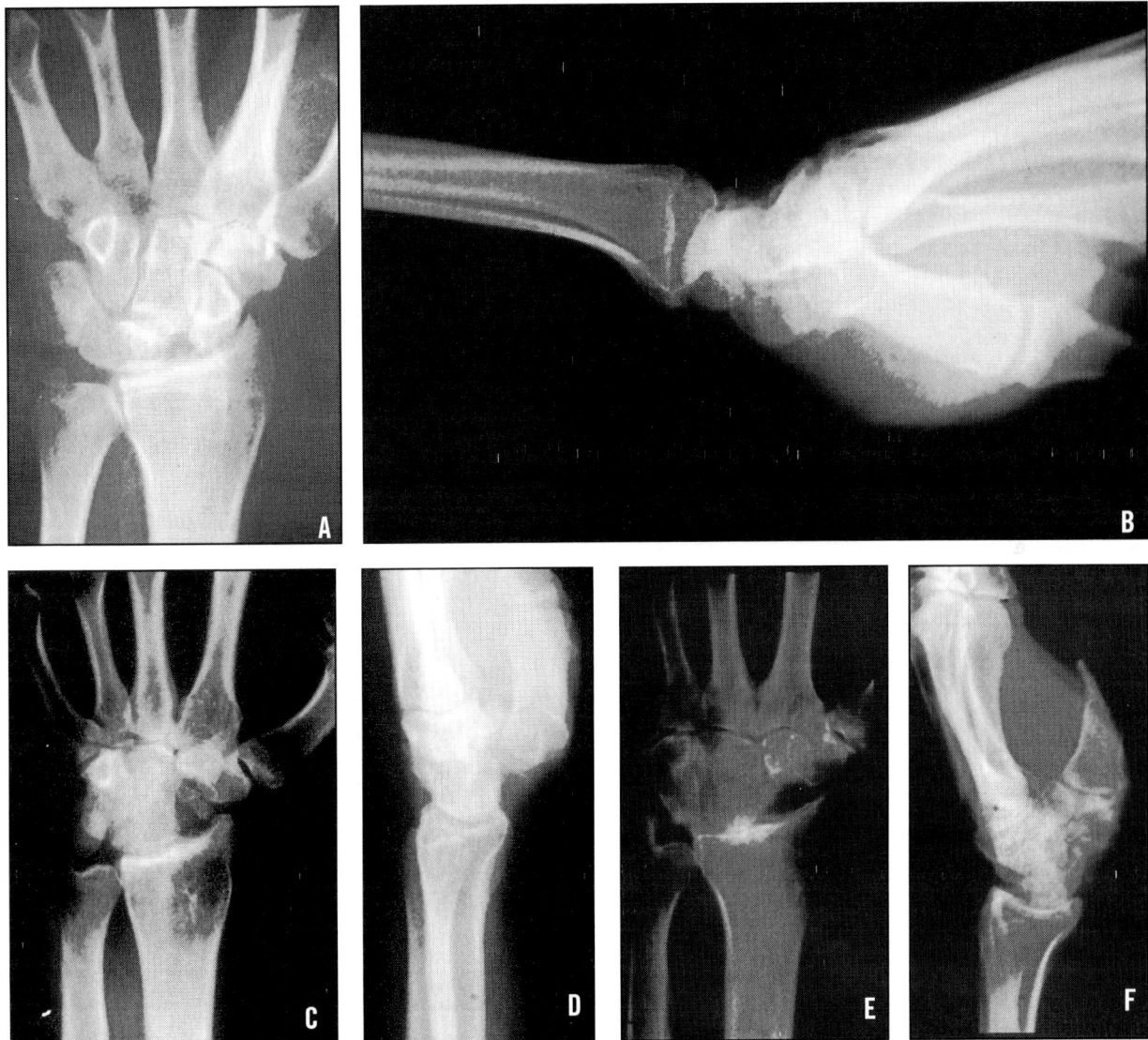

Wrist with a dorsal perilunate dislocation. PA (**A**) and lateral (**B**) radiographs show stage III SLAC arthritis 2 years following satisfactory early ORIF. Four-bone fusion and scaphoid excision (**C** and **D**) and PRC (**E** and **F**) are motion-preserving treatment options; when significant capitate arthrosis exists, the former is advised.

CONCLUSION

The late management of perilunate fracture-dislocations presents challenges. Delay in diagnosis exceeding 2 months may compromise the results of ORIF. Transient external fixation and distraction may facilitate atraumatic reduction, however. If articular cartilage on the capitate is relatively well maintained, PRC provides satisfactory pain relief and restores range of motion and grip strength, but wrist arthrodesis remains the definitive salvage procedure. When either ligamentous or osseous healing is incomplete and carpal instability complicates appropriate early treatment, the late development of SLAC arthritis may cause significant impairment. In such situations, PRC, intercarpal arthrodesis with scaphoid excision, and wrist fusion are effective alternatives.

REFERENCES

1. Kozin SH: Perilunate injuries: Diagnosis and treatment. *J Am Acad Orthop Surg* 1998;6:114-120.

2. Cooney WP, Bussey R, Dobyns JH, Linscheid RL: Difficult wrist fractures: Perilunate fracture-dislocations of the wrist. *Clin Orthop* 1987;214:136-147.

3. Herzberg G, Comtet JJ, Linscheid RL, Amadio PC, Cooney WP, Stalder J: Perilunate dislocations and fracture-dislocations: A multicenter study. *J Hand Surg Am* 1993;18: 768-779.

4. Ashmead D IV, Watson HK, Damon C, Herber S, Paly W: Scapholunate advanced collapse wrist salvage. *J Hand Surg Am* 1994;19:741-750.

5. Conyers DJ: Scapholunate interosseous reconstruction and imbrication of palmar ligaments. *J Hand Surg Am* 1990; 15:690-700.

6. Su CJ, Chang MC, Liu Y, Lo WH: Lunate and perilunate dislocation. *Zhonghua Yi Xue Za Zhi* 1996;58:348-354.

7. Howard FM, Dell PC: The unreduced carpal dislocation: A method of treatment. *Clin Orthop* 1986;202:112-116.

8. Vegter J: Late reduction of the dislocated lunate: A method using distraction by an external fixator. *J Bone Joint Surg Br* 1987;69:734-736.

9. Gellman H, Schwartz SD, Botte MJ, Feiwell L: Late treatment of a dorsal transscaphoid, transtriquetral perilunate wrist dislocation with avascular changes of the lunate. *Clin Orthop* 1988;237:196-203.

10. Siegert JJ, Frassica FJ, Amadio PC: Treatment of chronic perilunate dislocations. *J Hand Surg Am* 1988;13:206-212.

11. Weir IG: The late reduction of carpal dislocations. *J Hand Surg Br* 1992;17:137-139.

12. Inoue G, Shionoya K: Late treatment of unreduced perilunate dislocations. *J Hand Surg Br* 1999;24:221-225.

13. Rettig ME, Raskin KB: Long-term assessment of proximal row carpectomy for chronic perilunate dislocations. *J Hand Surg Am* 1999;24:1231-1236.

14. Tomaino MM, Miller RJ, Burton RI: Outcome assessment following limited wrist fusion: Objective wrist scoring versus patient satisfaction. *Contemp Orthop* 1994;28:403-410.

15. Palmer AK, Werner FW, Murphy D, Glisson R: Functional wrist motion: A biomechanical study. *J Hand Surg Am* 1985;10:39-46.

16. Shah J, Jones WA: Factors affecting the outcome in 50 cases of scaphoid nonunion treated with Herbert screw fixation. *J Hand Surg Br* 1998;23:680-685.

17. White RE Jr, Omer GE Jr: Transient vascular compromise of the lunate after fracture-dislocation or dislocation of the carpus. *J Hand Surg Am* 1984;9:181-184.

18. Linscheid RL, Dobyns JH, Beabout JW, Bryan RS: Traumatic instability of the wrist: Diagnosis, classification, and pathomechanics. *J Bone Joint Surg Am* 1972;54:1612-1632.

19. Tomaino MM, Delsignore J, Burton RI: Long-term results following proximal row carpectomy. *J Hand Surg Am* 1994;19:694-703.

20. Richards RS, Roth JH: Simultaneous proximal row carpectomy and radius to distal carpal row arthrodesis. *J Hand Surg Am* 1994;19:728-732.

21. Tomaino MM, Miller RJ, Cole I, Burton RI: Scapholunate advanced collapse wrist: Proximal row carpectomy or limited wrist arthrodesis with scaphoid excision? *J Hand Surg Am* 1994;19:134-142.

CHAPTER 9

POSTOPERATIVE REHABILITATION OF CARPAL DISLOCATIONS AND FRACTURE-DISLOCATIONS

JADE STRONG, MOT, OTR, CHT

MOLLY HUDSON, OTR, CHT

EVAN COLLINS, MD

Most serious carpal injuries are followed by some loss of range of motion, regardless of the method of treatment. However, appropriate and effective therapy can limit the amount of disability a patient sustains. This chapter presents a treatment algorithm to be used following surgery for fracture-dislocations or dislocations of the carpus.

Several basic principles should be followed in rehabilitating patients with these injuries. The first principle is to regard carpal stability as a priority. Various carpal surgical procedures accept some loss of range of motion as the price to be paid for achieving stability. The fact that stability is preferred over mobility should be kept in mind when determining the plan of care and treatment for each patient. Aggressive techniques such as stretching, used in an attempt to regain full range of motion at the risk of losing carpal stability, are not warranted. The second principle is to address the postoperative soft-tissue issues such as edema and stiffness that commonly accompany these injuries.

The rehabilitation of patients with surgically treated carpal dislocations or fracture-dislocations can be divided into three general phases. Phase one is the acute or initial phase of treatment, phase two can be considered the progressive phase, and phase three focuses on strengthening and conditioning. Each phase has its own potential pathologies and pitfalls that hand therapy can address. The timeline given should be regarded as a guideline only; physicians may need to adjust the duration of each phase depending on the surgical procedure performed. The condition of the structures involved may also influence when certain exercise protocols can be initiated. The physician should inform the hand therapist of any such concerns and should also communicate information about prognosis and acceptable outcomes with the therapist as well as the patient.

PHASE ONE

The initial phase of treatment begins immediately after surgery and lasts approximately 8 weeks. A soft, bulky compressive dressing is usually applied to the surgical site, along with a temporary splint that immobilizes the elbow in approximately 90° of flexion with the forearm and wrist in neutral and the thumb palmarly abducted; the interphalangeal (IP) joint is left mobilized. When present, edema or inflammation will occur during phase one. An inflammatory reaction usually accompanies these injuries and can last from 36 hours to 10 days after the injury.[1]

Casting

The patient returns to the office 7 to 10 days after surgery to have the dressing changed and a cast applied. Frequently, a long arm-thumb spica cast is used to stabilize the scaphoid. If appropriate for the type of injury, a Munster-type thumb spica cast is preferred; the Munster cast allows some flexion and extension of the elbow but prevents supination and pronation of the wrist; the joint of the thumb is left mobilized. The cast must be applied carefully to maintain the arches of the hand, making sure the distal end of the cast does not extend past the distal palmar crease. A cast that extends beyond that point usually blocks metacarpal motion, preventing full flexion at the metacarpophalangeal joint or keeping it in a nonphysiologic extended position. Exercises for active range of motion for both the shoulder and elbow and the fingers will be initiated while the patient is in the cast. During this phase, pain control is of paramount importance. The patient will remain in the long arm cast for approximately 4 weeks, after which a short arm cast is applied for an additional 4 weeks.[2]

Edema Control

Postoperative edema control is vital to minimize interstructural adhesions, joint stiffness, and pain. Edema can become a chronic problem if it is not addressed appropriately. The five techniques most commonly used for edema reduction during this first postoperative phase include elevation, ice, range-of-motion exercises, light compression, and high-voltage pulsed stimulation (HVPS).

Elevation After the immediate postoperative period, patients should be instructed in elevation of the upper extremity. The hand should be placed above the elbow, and the elbow should be higher than the level of the heart. Studies have shown that elevating the upper extremity 30° while in a supine position is effective in reducing edema. A patient who has been educated about how edema contributes to adhesions, fibrosis, and limited range of motion is more likely to comply with instructions to elevate the upper extremity.

Ice The application of a cold pack in the first 24 to 48 hours after onset of edema is often the treatment of choice. It is helpful in reducing not only edema but also pain in some patients.[3] Care must be exercised when applying cold to the affected extremity. Lievens and Leduc[4] found that extreme temperatures may actually increase edema because of increased permeability of the lymph vessels. This is seen at about 15° C. When application of cold is prescribed, the patient must be properly educated regarding monitoring of vascular status and about frequency, duration, and methods of application.

Range-of-Motion Exercises Range-of-motion exercises have dual benefits. They not only maintain digital range of motion but also, in the initial phases of healing, act as a pump to decrease any edema that may have accumulated in the fingers. The patient should be instructed to perform 20 repetitions of overhead fisting every hour. The active fist (volitional opening and closing of the hand) must be made forcefully enough to result in blanching of

the metacarpals but not so forcefully as to create a loading force on the carpus. The IP joints must be flexed and extended throughout the entire arc of motion. Wiggling of the fingers will not produce blanching and therefore is not effective in propelling fluids out of the fingers.[3]

Compression Light compression has been documented to effectively reduce edema.[5] Compressive techniques include string wrapping, self-adhesive elastic wrapping, and compressive gloves.[3] Both the string and the self-adhesive elastic wrap must always be applied from distal to proximal, paying careful attention to the tension; if the wrapping is too tight, it can restrict circulation. These techniques should be performed initially by the therapist and then carefully taught to the patient to maximize compliance and reduce the risk of complications.

High-Voltage Pulsed Stimulation HVPS, also called galvanic stimulation, is a type of interrupted monophasic wave-form stimulation. The physiologic theory behind HVPS therapy is that with acute edema, proteins leak into interstitial spaces; the electric current of HVPS forces the proteins to move into the lymphatic system, away from the interstitial spaces.[3] HVPS has been shown clinically to reduce edema. Unfortunately, the US Food and Drug Administration does not recognize edema reduction and wound healing as benefits of HVPS, despite the fact that numerous studies have shown significant improvements in these areas with the use of HVPS.[6] The recommended HVPS parameters for treating acute edema are as follows: negative polarity; high frequency (approximately 80 to 100 pulses per second); continuous mode; sensory-only intensity (no muscle contraction); and duration of 15 to 30 minutes four times per day.

Circumferential stimulation is often preferred for the hand; however, this may be difficult to achieve in the acute phase because of the bulky postoperative dressing or long arm cast. One approach is to wrap the exposed fingers collectively with gel-impregnated cold wrap dressings and attach a large ground electrode to the proximal upper extremity (Fig. 1). The edema reduction techniques described here all have been shown to be effective in isolation. However, using them in combination will produce the optimal result.

Stiffness of Uninvolved Joints

An important concern but one that is frequently overlooked is preserving function in structures and joints adjacent to the injured wrist. Huffaker and associates[7] found that 29% of patients in a large series experienced a decrease in range of motion of the uninvolved fingers

FIGURE 1

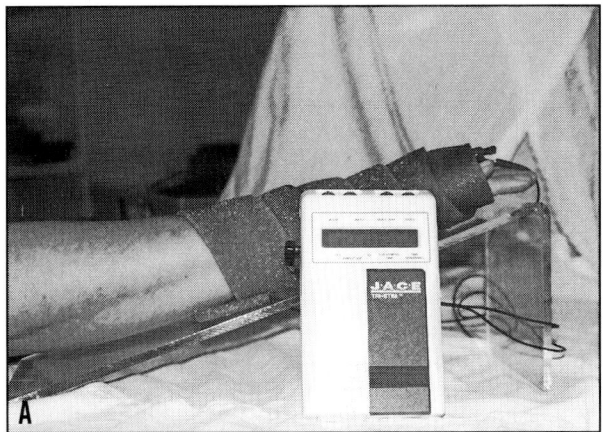

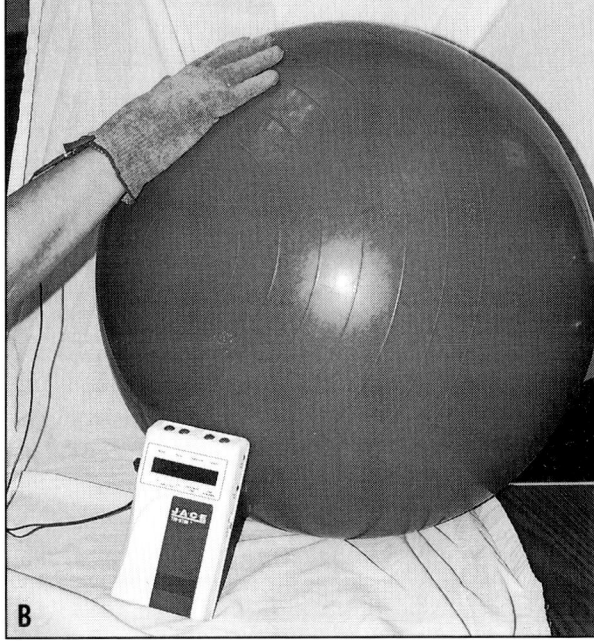

Edema reduction techniques used in combination. **A,** HVPS used in conjunction with gel-impregnated cold wrap and elevation. **B,** HVPS used in conjunction with a compression glove and elevation.

and hand following a fracture of the hand. Active range of motion and function of the fingers should never be ignored because the wrist will not function properly if the adjacent structures have diminished function. Thus, range-of-motion exercises for the elbow, shoulder, and hand in their available planes of motion should be started as soon as the patient can tolerate them.

To address finger stiffness, a three-part approach is recommended. First, it is important to determine whether the stiffness is caused by continued edema or by failure to maintain motion. Edema should be treated with ice, light compressive dressings, elevation, and manual edema mobilization. Second, while the patient is still in the cast, active assisted range-of-motion exercises are extremely important. The danger of aggressive passive range-of-motion exercises is that they may stress patients beyond their pain limits, resulting in more edema. This invokes a negative feedback cycle that can initiate more stiffness or scar tissue or, as has been reported,[8] a reflex sympathetic dystrophy. Unfortunately, no objective measurement is available to help the therapist judge the amount of force that should be applied with active assisted range of motion. The therapist must decide this by gauging the patient's level of pain and the "end-feel" and heat of the joint,[9] avoiding tearing the tissues and thus creating an inflammatory response.[10] Recommended active and active assisted range-of-motion exercises include joint blocking, tendon gliding, and place and hold exercises. Joint blocking allows for isolated flexor digitorum superficialis and flexor digitorum profundus excursion. Active tendon gliding exercises allow for differential glide of intrinsic and extrinsic tendons. These have been shown to be effective in improving or maintaining digital range of motion during this phase. Place and hold exercises, which are based on extensive studies of tendon trauma, may be helpful in the case of limited active range of motion or weakness.[11] Place and hold is performed by passively placing the fingers in the direction of deficit and asking the patient to hold the position while the passive pressure is released. Early introduction of these range-of-motion exercises helps to manage scar tissue adhesions of extrinsic tendons that cross the carpal region. Optimal results seem to occur when exercises are performed frequently throughout the day rather than in one long session. If approved by the physician, submaximal isometric exercises of the wrist muscles may be initiated to assist in prevention and reduction of muscle atrophy. Finally, light prehension activities and functional tasks without resistance (eg, nuts and bolts) are encouraged. Special attention to preserving joint range of motion should be paid to patients with arthritic changes in the hand.

PHASE TWO

Phase two usually lasts from approximately 8 to 16 weeks after surgery. It begins when the splint or cast has been either discontinued or is being used only intermittently. Any Kirschner wires used in surgery are usually removed

8 weeks postoperatively.[2] This rehabilitation phase should be initiated only when adequate wrist stability has been achieved. Physical deficits that may be experienced during this phase include wrist and forearm stiffness, scar tissue or adhesions, mechanical dysfunction, and muscle weakness. In addition, if finger stiffness or edema persist from phase one, treatment may need to be modified accordingly by the therapist.

Wrist and Forearm Stiffness

Immobilization for any length of time can have a devastating effect on range of motion. To prevent wrist and forearm stiffness, stretching and passive range-of-motion exercises may be indicated during stage two. The therapist should be careful not to disrupt the repair or to over-mobilize either the involved or uninvolved joints. Wrist stiffness can be addressed using a variety of therapeutic techniques such as active range of motion, nonresistive functional tasks, and thermal modalities.

Heat Superficial heating agents, such as the moist hot pack, produce maximum heat at a depth of 0.5 cm in 6 to 8 minutes. Lower levels of heat may be obtained at a depth of 1 to 2 cm with prolonged exposure of 15 to 30 minutes and may be beneficial.[12] Superficial heat is associated with an increase in blood flow to the skin, while positive vascular effects are seen in skeletal muscle in response to an increase in exercise level.[13] Recommendations for the use of heat in patients who have undergone surgery for carpal fracture-dislocations include applying heat prior to exercise for 15 to 20 minutes, followed by active exercise. Combining low-load stretching and heat produces greater benefits than heat alone.

Ultrasound Ultrasound is a high-frequency acoustic energy used in rehabilitation programs to restore mobility, reduce pain, and enhance tissue healing. It elevates tissue temperatures at a depth of 3 to 5 cm without creating excessive heat in the superficial structures.[14] The physiologic advantages of ultrasound include increased collagen tissue extensibility, blood flow, pain threshold, and enzymatic activity and alteration of nerve conduction velocity. At this phase of rehabilitation, ultrasound is used to alter the viscoelastic properties of collagen tissue and molecular bonding to facilitate easier range of motion.[14] Ultrasound was found to be more effective when active range-of-motion exercises followed the ultrasound treatment.[15] The therapist applying ultrasound should fully understand its principles, indications, and contraindications. General guidelines for the use of ultrasound following wrist surgery are as follows: intensity of 0.8 to 1.5 W/cm^2; 1 or 3 MHz;

continuous wave or 20% for 5 to 8 minutes; a total of 12 to 15 treatments, depending on the location and presence and severity of edema. These parameters may need to be adjusted depending on how frequently the patient is seen (eg, overuse causing an increase in edema may indicate using a pulsed-duty rather than continuous-wave cycle).

Splinting If functional active range of motion of the wrist is restricted, dynamic, static-progressive, or serial splinting to improve range of motion may be used at this stage. The physician must verify that the fractures are healed prior to the initiation of aggressive splinting. Flexion splinting should be avoided if the surgical procedure involved creating a dorsal checkrein. Wrist splints are usually implemented to remodel scar adhesions. The basis for this is the assertion that the stretch represents a passive action that in turn results in tissue elongation.[10] It is critical to avoid stretching to the point of rupture, which would result in inflammation and further scar formation. To achieve true lengthening, a low-load static progressive stretch must be applied. This allows old collagen to be absorbed and new collagen to be laid down. For wrists with a hard end-feel, a static progressive splint, which is most effective in creating plastic deformation and therefore lengthening the tissues, is preferred.[16] The design of a static progressive splint includes a customized orthoplast molded circumferentially around the forearm and ending proximal to the wrist crease. A hand-based splint with the thumb and fingers mobilized is fabricated around the hand with an inelastic monofilament line attached to the dorsum of the splint. The monofilament line runs directly to the static progressive component that is attached to the dorsum of the forearm splint. A thumb-screw on the static progressive component is used to adjust the tension. The splint maintains the wrist tissue in a position of extension (or flexion) near the end of the elastic limit, with the ultimate goal of tissue lengthening.

Active Range of Motion

Active range-of-motion exercises initiated in phase one (ie, tendon gliding exercises, joint blocking, place and hold exercises) should be continued in this phase as needed to address limitations in digital range of motion.

Medical Exercise Training Medical exercise training (MET) is a series of exercises that involve several repetitions of a short arc of pain-free, active motion. MET is based on the Holton curve, which determines the particular dosage, repetition, and rest periods most appropriate for a patient's specific needs. Unloaded METs are beneficial in the early stages of rehabilitation because they increase the nutrient supply and eliminate by-product waste caused by the inflammatory process through improved blood flow. Unloaded METs are performed for 2 to 5 minutes in each wrist plane of motion, including flexion-extension, ulnar-radial deviation, and pronation-supination. These exercises may be performed as often as every hour as long as swelling does not increase. If this occurs, exercise frequency may be reduced from every 2 hours to three times per day. METs have been observed clinically to reduce pain and therefore are helpful in preparation for performing functional tasks (P Sizer, MS, PT, Amarillo, TX, unpublished data, 2000).

Functional Tasks Functional or purposeful activity tasks should always be incorporated into therapeutic intervention. Purposeful activities are activities with an inherent goal that is relevant to the patient,[17] as determined by the patient. They can include any bilateral activity that involves multiple joints and motor patterns and is appropriate and important to the patient's activities of daily living, either vocational or avocational. Tasks that provide tangible and meaningful outcomes, such as an auto mechanic disassembling and assembling a small carburetor, seem to be more rewarding.

Edema

If edema persists into the second phase of rehabilitation, the cause of the edema should be reassessed. Additional reduction techniques might be tried, such as HVPS on a lower frequency setting or manual edema mobilization. If a compressive dressing is being used during this phase and the patient reports increased swelling while wearing the dressing, excessive pressure from the dressing may be causing a collapse of the distal lymphatic system, trapping fluid in the interstitial region. If this occurs, the pressure dressings must be discontinued and the approach reassessed.

HVPS During phase two, the HVPS described for phase one can be used but with parameters that target chronic edema. Recommended settings for chronic edema may include[15] negative polarity, a low frequency of 20 to 30 pulses per second, and a duration of 20 minutes, three times per day.

Manual Edema Mobilization Manual edema mobilization as described by Artzberger (SM Artzberger, OTR, New Orleans, LA, unpublished data, 1998) is a form of light massage that uses "clear" and "flow" techniques to stimulate lymphatic flow. It has been shown clinically to reduce edema effectively. Manual edema mobilization

should be performed only by a trained therapist. Further discussion of this technique and its effectiveness is beyond the scope of this chapter.

Scar Tissue

Ultrasound Ultrasound not only has a definite role in providing a deep thermal heat but is also used to restore mobility when scarring is present. Although many therapists use ultrasound in the belief that it actually decreases scar formation, the results of studies on this use of ultrasound have been inconclusive. Often, surgery to the wrist can cause a length restriction of the joint capsules or prevent smooth gliding of the soft tissues.[18,19] Bierman[20] administered ultrasound to patients with scar tissue from X-rays, lacerations, and Dupuytren's contracture and found it successfully increased the range of motion in all patients. However, this increase in range of motion is believed to be due to an increase in the elasticity of the scar tissue as a result of the heat of the ultrasound. Because scar tissue is denser than surrounding tissues, ultrasound selectively heats the scar tissue prior to scar massage and range-of-motion exercises, thereby facilitating scar elongation.

Massage Both clinical and experimental trials have demonstrated that biomechanical changes within tissue that occur with scarring have a negative effect on function. Scar management involves various techniques such as active range of motion, applied controlled stress (ie, static progressive splinting), scar pads, and soft-tissue mobilization. Such techniques do not actually break up scar tissue but increase the pliability and facilitate elongation of the tissues. Deep transverse friction massage that crosses the grain of the connective tissue is applied to mobilize the superficial scar by stretching its underlying tissue adhesions. Heat and ultrasound applied prior to the massage increase the elasticity of the tissues, thereby increasing the effectiveness of the massage.[19]

Scar Mold or Pad A bulky, superficial scar can be treated with a scar mold or pad made of elastomer, prosthetic foam, or silicone sheeting. The mold or pad provides continuous pressure, resulting in a flatter, softer scar that is more elastic and cosmetically appealing. The mold or pad should be worn as continuously as possible without impeding functional motion. Although the effectiveness of the scar pad has been demonstrated clinically, some reports consider the effects short-lived, the result of dehydration and mechanical effects of compression.[21] Because scar bulk cannot be measured reliably, research remains inconclusive in this area.

FIGURE 2

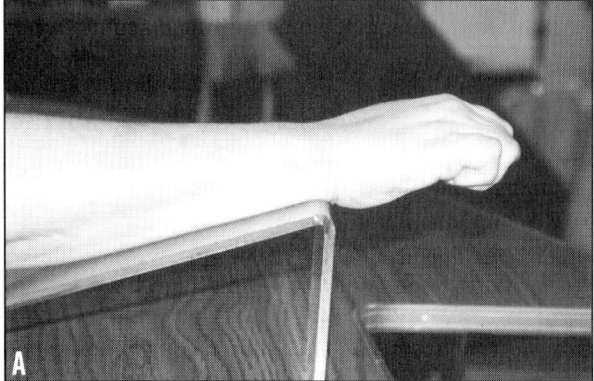

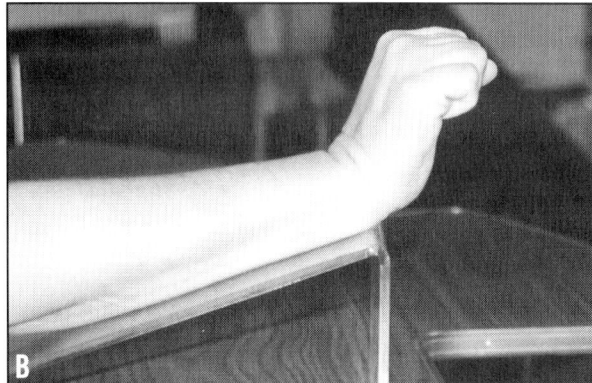

Muscle reeducation techniques. **A,** Improper wrist extension using extensor digitorum communis as a compensatory technique. **B,** Correct use of extensor carpi radialis brevis/longus and extensor carpi ulnaris.

FIGURE 3

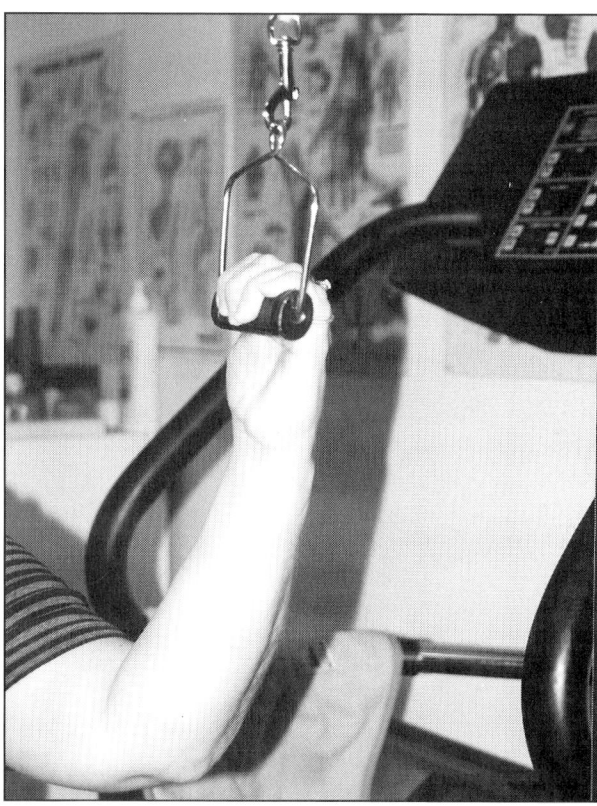

Hanging exercise. The wrist is in neutral, producing a co-contraction of the wrist flexors and extensors.

Mechanical Dysfunction

Dysfunction can occur with an imbalance in proper wrist biomechanics in the bone, ligament, or musculotendinous unit. Such dysfunction can be addressed therapeutically without placing increased stress on the carpus.

Muscle Reeducation Immobilization of the wrist for a prolonged period of time can create weakness and impaired coordination. Muscle reeducation techniques include any forms of exercise that isolate the active wrist flexors and extensors. The patient should focus on contracting the wrist muscles without involving accessory muscles or using compensatory techniques (ie, using the extensor digitorum communis greater than the extensor carpi radialis brevis/longus and extensor carpi ulnaris) (Fig. 2). Place and hold techniques are helpful in reducing compensatory patterns and providing proprioceptive feedback. In one type of place and hold exercise, the therapist places the patient's fingers in a fisted position and

the wrist in extension and asks the patient to hold the position to the best of his or her ability. The therapist then releases the passive pressure. Place and hold exercises may be modified as appropriate for limited active wrist flexion or forearm pronation and supination. Other proprioceptive exercises may be helpful after a prolonged period of immobilization.

Hanging Another technique that may improve wrist mechanics is the hanging program (P Sizer, MEd, PT, International Academy of Orthopaedic Medicine, unpublished data, 2000). The purpose of this program is to create a stabilizing force across the carpus by co-contraction of the wrist flexors and extensors and the long finger flexors without creating excessive force to the carpus. The exercises are initiated with the patient holding onto an overhead pulley system using the hook grasp (intrinsic minus) position (Fig. 3). The hook grasp (metacarpal phalangeal joints extended; proximal interphalangeal/distal

FIGURE 4

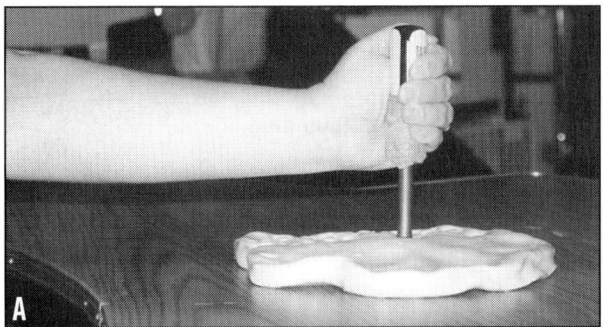

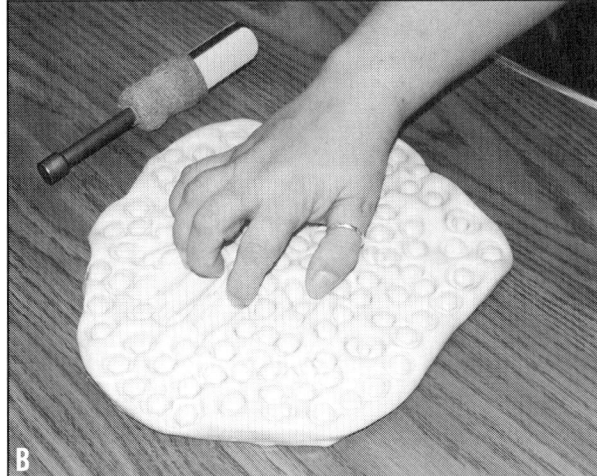

Isometric exercises using resistive putty. **A,** Putty punch exercise. **B,** Putty drag exercise.

interphalangeal joints in full flexion) is used to prevent the lumbricals from migrating proximally into the carpal canal and the lunate from translating onto the capitate.[22] Maintaining the wrist in neutral, the patient pulls, using approximately 30% of his or her maximum volitional contraction. This isometric position is held for 90 seconds and alternated with 30-second rest periods. This 3:1 ratio of on to off time is maintained, but the number of repetitions and and percent of maximum volitional contraction can vary depending on the patient's range of motion, pain level, and strength, with a typical regimen being 10 repetitions three times a day. This program was developed based on well-accepted studies and is felt to be of clinical significance, though further scientific studies are needed.

Weakness

Submaximal Isometric Exercises Isometric exercises involve the application of force or muscle contraction

without actual movement occurring. Isometric training strengthens only at the specific joint angle at which the exercise is performed and does not improve the ability to exert force rapidly. The benefits of isometric exercise are usually obtained during the early stages of rehabilitation. Muscle contraction is kept submaximal to prevent overloading the carpus yet allow for recruitment of muscle fiber to assist in reeducating the muscles and slowing the atrophy process. Following wrist surgery, isometric exercises are recommended prior to isotonic exercises. One example of an isometric exercise is pressing a minimally resistant 20-oz putty flat against a hard surface. Once the putty is flattened, a nut driver or BTE (Baltimore Therapeutic Equipment Company, Inc, Baltimore, MD) attachment 502 or 504 is pressed into the putty in rows to create a "waffle" effect. The patient then hooks his or her fingers into the putty with the wrist in neutral and drags the putty toward the patient (Fig. 4). Partial grip strengthening using a gripper provides isotonic exercise for the digital flexors and an isometric exercise through the wrist.

PHASE THREE

Phase three begins approximately 12 to 16 weeks after surgery. During this phase, resistive strengthening exercises are introduced after range of motion within functional limits is attained.[23] The patient's status and goals must be considered when choosing appropriate exercises. In establishing treatments and home programs, the therapist should consider the demands that the patient will be placing on the upper extremity to achieve the goals of mobility, strength, endurance, dexterity, and flexibility. During early strengthening phases, caution should be taken to avoid forceful closed grip activity to prevent both proximal migration of the lumbricals into the carpal region, creating an increase in pressure, and loading of the lunate onto the capitate.[22] Holton's curve is helpful in developing individualized exercise programs and determining specific dosage to achieve goals (J Wagenbrenner, PT, Seattle, WA, unpublished data, 1997). Furthermore, the concept of "no pain, no gain" is not the rule in this case. Patient reports of pain should be monitored closely and treatment modified as indicated.

Strengthening

Isometric Strengthening Isometric strengthening, which has been found to be one of the most effective methods of strengthening (J Wagenbrenner, PT, Seattle, WA, unpublished data, 1997), is static in that target muscles stay a con-

FIGURE 5

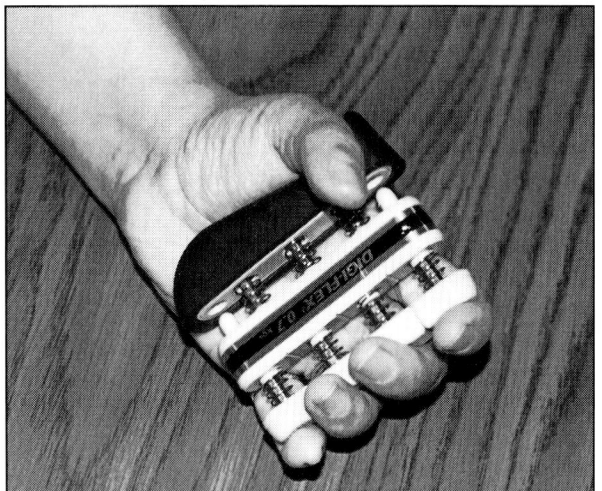

Patient using a finger exerciser with spring-loaded buttons.

FIGURE 6

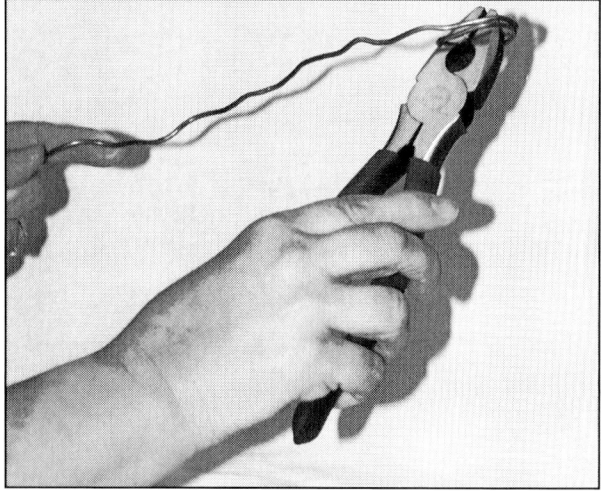

Patient performing the functional task of curling 1/8-in copper wire with pliers. The task requires a strong grip, good active range of motion, and sustained endurance.

stant length. Examples of isometric training of the wrist extensor are the "putty punch and drag" described previously and bicep curls while holding a dumbbell with the wrist in slight extension. Grip strengthening also helps the patient isolate the target muscles when performing isometric co-contractions of the wrist flexors and extensors and dynamic work to the long finger flexors.

Grip Strengthening For the most effective grip strengthening, Lindsay (M Lindsay, PT, San Francisco, CA, unpublished data, 1991) recommends the following four types of training: eccentric, rapid twitch, interval training, and simulated functional tasks. Eccentric grip strengthening concentrates on the slow lengthening phase, when the "muscle is controlling the motion." This type of training adds muscle bulk and increases strength. Rapid twitch training involves low resistance at high repetition. This may be achieved using a finger exerciser with spring-loaded buttons, instructing the patient to perform 100 repetitions as quickly as possible without pain (Fig. 5). Resistance should be such that fatigue occurs toward the end of the set. Although rapid twitch fibers are important to functional coordination and endurance, they are often neglected. Interval training develops strength by promoting the depletion and replenishing of oxygen. This training involves maintaining a contraction for 60 seconds at approximately 75% to 85% of maximum grip, followed by a rest period of 60 seconds. This exercise is repeated 3 to 15 times, depending on the patient's needs. The last type of training involves performing functional tasks determined by the patient's needs and goals, such as open-

ing jars or using woodworking tools. These tasks should be individualized to the patient's needs and should incorporate functional motor patterns. The combination of these four exercises have been shown clinically to maximize the successful return to premorbid functioning.

Wrist Strengthening Several forms of dynamic wrist strengthening are performed during stage three. The focus is on eccentric lengthening because it requires half the amount of energy that a concentric contraction requires, thus allowing twice the amount of work to be done for the same energy expenditure. Resistive tubing or dumbbells may be used. With the goals of improving circulation, developing coordination, and increasing endurance, Holton recommends starting at 60% of the patient's maximum one-repetition lift with three sets of 24 repetitions and a 30-second break between sets. If pain or hypermobility is an issue, these exercises should be performed in the midrange of motion (J Wagenbrenner, PT, Seattle, WA, unpublished data, 1997). Again, incorporating functional tasks, such as using a screwdriver or pliers, is encouraged (Fig. 6).

Muscle Reeducation Muscle reeducation is described earlier, in phases one and two, but sometimes these exercises need to be continued. The hanging program may be continued, with resistance increased to 80% of perceived maximal effort and with a 2:1 ratio of rest to contraction. In cases of extreme weakness and adhesions, electrical stimulation may be helpful.

FIGURE 7

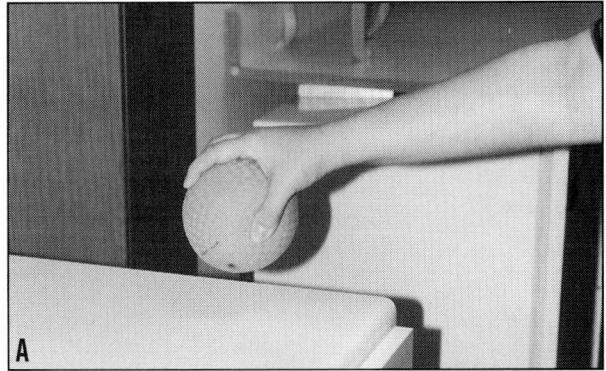

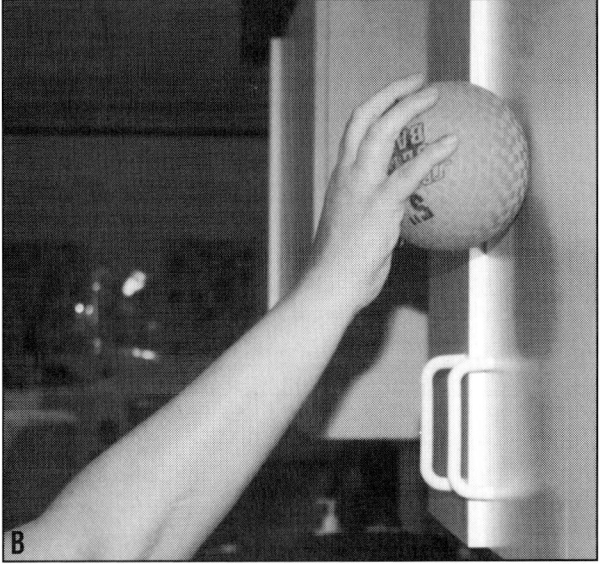

Exercises using a weighted ball. **A,** The patient bounces the ball against a horizontal surface. **B,** In this more advanced exercise, the ball is bounced against a vertical surface.

Advanced Training Exercises Dynamic stabilization, plyometrics, and weight bearing should be incorporated once the patient has demonstrated an increase in static and dynamic muscle work without pain. These exercises can be performed in several different positions and motor patterns to alter the level of difficulty. Exercises using a weighted ball against a vertical surface, horizontal surface, or rebound trampoline are helpful in training acceleration and deceleration of forearm and upper quadrant muscles (Fig. 7). These advanced exercises require quick grasp and release with good wrist stabilization. Weight bearing should be performed only when the patient is completely pain free. This may progress from wall push-ups to floor

push-ups and push-ups using a therapeutic ball. It is especially important to incorporate these exercises into the rehabilitation of active individuals, but they must be approved by the physician.

A work conditioning or work hardening program should be considered if a patient is returning to manual labor after a prolonged period of restricted duty or off work in order to facilitate a successful return to work. Work conditioning is separate from the rehabilitation in that it uses work-oriented tasks to build endurance, strength, and productivity levels. Psychosocial and psychological issues related to the injury such as pain and reduced confidence may be addressed at this level as well. Work conditioning after a wrist injury should include work-simulated tasks tailored for the individual patient's needs. Commercially produced work simulators and assembly boards are useful tools, though therapists should not rely solely on these tools. Therapists should use creativity in developing a patient's program to promote motivation and to facilitate a successful return to work.[24]

CONCLUSION

The ultimate goal of rehabilitation after wrist surgery is achieving a stable and pain-free joint that has sufficient mobility and strength to enable the patient to return to the previous level of activity. The treatments described in this chapter are most beneficial to the patient when they are closely monitored and adjusted when appropriate. Too quick a progression can disrupt the surgical repair, thus delaying or impeding the healing process and possibly leading to a poor outcome. In addition, recovery will vary depending on the age of the patient, the severity of the injury, and the surgical repair. Therefore, all of these factors must be considered when developing a treatment program.

REFERENCES

1. Davidson JM: Wound repair. *J Hand Ther* 1998;11:80-94.
2. Cohen M, Talesnik J: Direct ligament repair of scapholunate dissociation with capsular augmentation. Advanced Techniques for the Treatment of Carpal Instabilities. Postgraduate conference by the American Society for Surgery of the Hand. Seattle, WA, October, 2000.
3. Hunter JM, Mackin E: Edema: Techniques of evaluation and management, in Hunter JM, Mackin E, Callahan AD (eds): *Rehabilitation of the Hand: Surgery and Therapy,* ed 4. St Louis, MO, Mosby-Year Book, 1995.

4. Lievens P, Leduc A: Cryotherapy and sports. *Int J Sports Med* 1984;5(suppl):37-39.

5. Flowers K: Abstract: String wrapping versus massage for reducing digital volume. *J Hand Surg Am* 1985;10:583.

6. Bettany JA, Fish DR, Mendel FC: High-voltage pulsed direct current: Effect on edema formation after hyperflexion injury. *Arch Phys Med Rehabil* 1990;71:677-681.

7. Huffaker WH, Wray RC Jr, Weeks PM: Factors influencing final range of motion in the fingers after fractures of the hand. *Plast Reconstr Surg* 1979;63:82-87.

8. Lankford LL: Reflex sympathetic dystrophy, in Hunter JM, Mackin E, Callahan AD (eds): *Rehabilitation of the Hand: Surgery and Therapy,* ed 4. St Louis, MO, Mosby-Year Book, 1995.

9. Merritt WH: Written on behalf of the stiff finger. *J Hand Ther* 1998;11:74-79.

10. Brand PW, Hollister A (eds): *Clinical Mechanics of the Hand,* ed 2. St Louis, MO, Mosby-Year Book, 1993.

11. Trumble TE, Sailer SM: Flexor tendon injuries, in Trumble TE (ed): *Principles of Hand Surgery and Therapy.* Philadelphia, PA, WB Saunders, 2000, pp 231-262.

12. Abramson DI, Mitchell RE, Tuck S Jr, Bell Y, Zayas AM: Changes in blood flow, oxygen uptake and tissue temperatures produced by the topical application of wet heat. *Arch Phys Med Rehabil* 1961;42:305-318.

13. Crockford GW, Hellon RF: Vascular responses of human skin to infra-red radiation. *J Physiol* 1959;149:424-432.

14. Ziskin MC, McDiarmid T, Michlovitz SL: Therapeutic ultrasound, in Michlovitz SL (ed): *Thermal Agents in Rehabilitation,* ed 2. Philadelphia, PA, FA Davis, 1990, pp 134-169.

15. Lehmann JF, McMillan JA, Brunner GD, Blumberg JB: Comparative study of the efficiency of short-wave, microwave and ultrasonic diathermy in heating the hip joint. *Arch Phys Med Rehabil* 1959;40:510-512.

16. Fess EE, Philips CA (eds): *Hand Splinting: Principles and Methods,* ed 2. St Louis, MO, CV Mosby, 1987.

17. Ayres AJ: Basic concepts of clinical practice in physical disabilities. *Am J Occup Ther* 1958;12:300-302.

18. Watson N: What is stiffness? *J Hand Ther* 1994;7:147-149.

19. Michlovitz SL: Use of ultrasound in upper extremity rehabilitation, in Hunter JM, Mackin E, Callahan AD (eds): *Rehabilitation of the Hand: Surgery and Therapy,* ed 4. St Louis, MO, Mosby-Year Book, 1995.

20. Bierman W: Ultrasound in the treatment of scars. *Arch Phys Med Rehabil* 1954;35:209-214.

21. Sullivan J: Abstract: Scar management techniques with the use of pressure contact dressings postreconstructive surgery. *J Hand Surg Am* 1984;9:610.

22. Viegas SF, Patterson R, Peterson P, Roefs J, Tencer A, Choi S: The effects of various load paths and different loads on the load transfer characteristics of the wrist. *J Hand Surg Am* 1989;14:458-465.

23. Andrews JR, Harrelson GL: *Physical Rehabilitation of the Injured Athlete.* Philadelphia, PA, WB Saunders, 1991.

24. Schultz-Johnson K: Work hardening and work conditioning, in Hunter JM, Mackin E, Callahan AD (eds): *Rehabilitation of the Hand: Surgery and Therapy,* ed 4. St Louis, MO, Mosby-Year Book, 1995.

INDEX